Johnson's®

breastfeeding

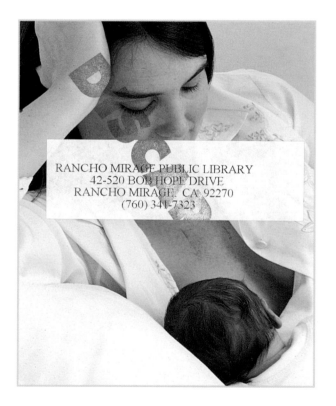

London, New York, Munich, Melbourne, Delhi

Text by Joanna Moorhead
For Rosie, Elinor, Miranda, and Catriona

Senior editor Julia North
U.S. senior editor Jennifer Williams
Senior art editors Glenda Fisher, Hannah Moore
Project editor Angela Baynham
Project art editor Alison Tumer
DTP designer Karen Constanti
Production controller Heather Hughes
Managing editor Anna Davidson
Managing art editor Emma Forge
Photography art direction Sally Smallwood
Photography Ruth Jenkinson
Americanizer Christine Heilman
Proofreader Lucas Mansell

Category publisher Corinne Roberts

First American Edition, 2004
Published in the United States by
DK Publishing, Inc.
375 Hudson Street
New York, New York 10014

03 04 05 06 07 08 10 9 8 7 6 5 4 3 2 1

A Cataloging-in-Publication record for this book is available from the Library of Congress.
ISBN 0-7566-0354-4
Reproduced by Colourscan
Printed in Italy by Graphicom

Discover more at
www.dk.com

A message to parents from

Johnson's®

The most precious gift in the world is a new baby. To your little one, you are the center of the universe. And by following your most basic instincts to touch, hold, and talk to your baby, you provide the best start to a happy, healthy life.

Our baby products encourage parents to care for and nurture their children through the importance of touch, developing a deep, loving bond that transcends all others.

Parenting is not an exact science, nor is it a one-size-fits-all formula. For more than a hundred years, Johnson & Johnson has supported the healthcare needs of parents and healthcare professionals, and we understand that all parents feel more confident in their role when they have information they can trust.

That is why we offer this book as our commitment to you to provide scientifically sound, professionally reviewed guidance on the important topics of pregnancy, babycare, and child development.

As you read through this book, the most important thing to remember is this: you know your baby better than anyone else. By watching, listening, and having confidence in your natural ability, you will know how to use the information you have in your hands, for the benefit of the baby in your arms.

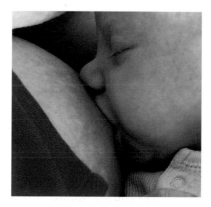

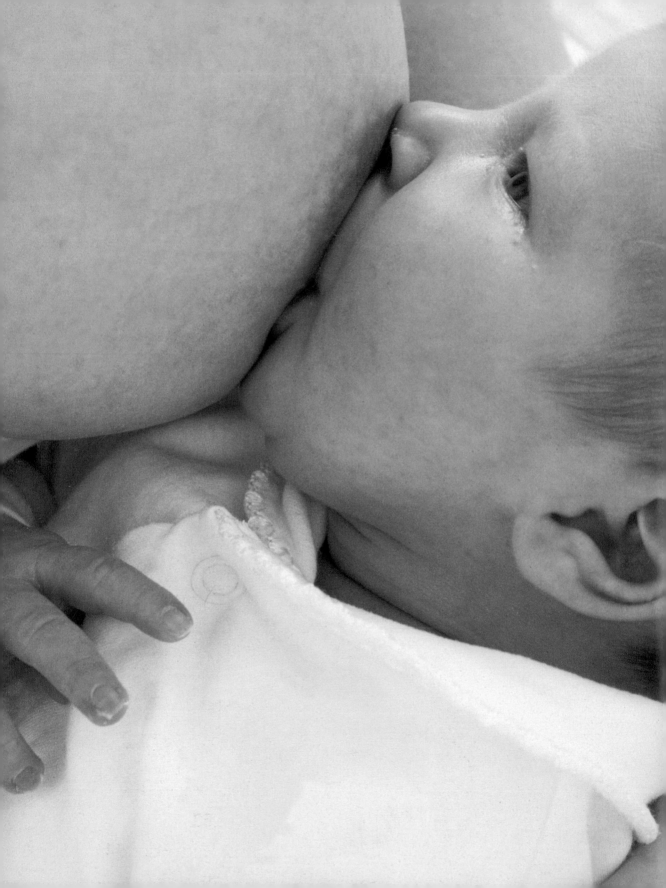

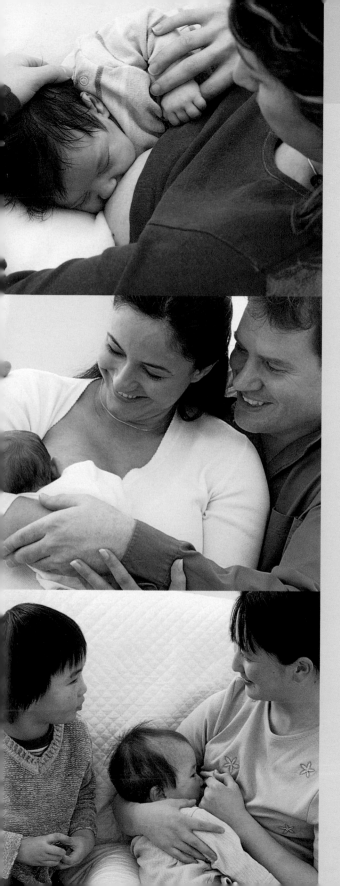

Contents

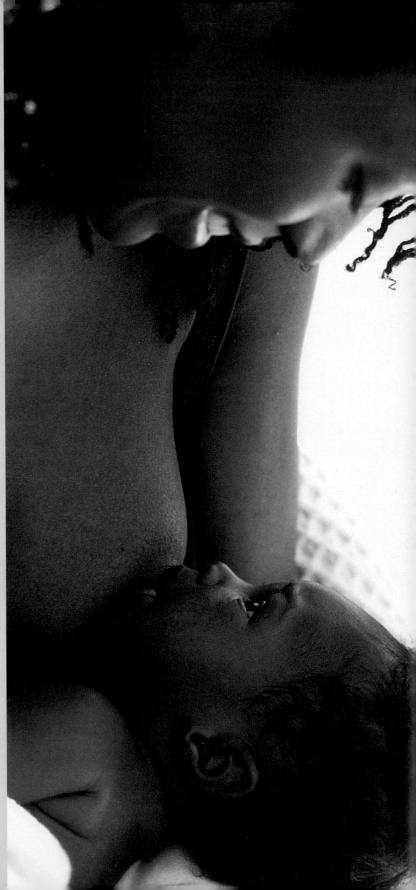

" Ben is a gorgeous, healthy baby—he **positively glows** with health. I love watching him at the breast and thinking to myself, that's **pure goodness.** "

ELLEN, mother of six-week-old Ben

1

The benefits of breastfeeding

Breastfeeding will give your baby the best possible start in life. Wherever you are, whatever your circumstances, whether you've given birth to a full-term baby or one who is premature—breastfeeding is a gift that's yours, and yours alone, to give to your child.

Benefits for your baby

Breast milk is the perfect food for your baby because it has been developed and designed over thousands of years with him in mind. However good formula milk is—and it's true to say that it is better now than it's ever been—it can at best only mimic breast milk, and will never be as good as the real thing. Why? Because breast milk is packed with the exact nutrients a human baby needs. It also contains living antibodies from your body that help protect your baby from disease.

For hundreds of years, all over the world, people have understood that breast milk protects babies as well as helping them to grow. Over recent years, doctors and scientists have carried out studies to show exactly how strong the protection offered by breast milk is, and more studies are being carried out all the time. These studies have all reached the same conclusion: breastfeeding protects your child against illness, both in the first few months of life and during the childhood years beyond.

• Breastfed babies are at far lower risk of gastrointestinal illnesses, which are responsible for the hospitalization of a sizable number of babies every year.

• Exclusive breastfeeding protects against respiratory illness: one study found that babies fed by bottle, or combined breast and bottle, ran twice the risk of getting a lung or respiratory tract infection of some kind.

• Urinary tract infections are less common among breastfed babies; bottle-fed babies were found to be at five times higher risk of these.

• Ear infections are less common among breastfed babies.

• Studies suggest that breastfeeding also offers some protection against Sudden Infant Death Syndrome (SIDS).

Research results

Studies show that breastfed babies reach their milestones quicker than other babies.

In particular, they seem to:

• learn to crawl earlier

• learn to speak sooner

• have a higher IQ—babies breastfed for between seven and nine months have higher intelligence on average than those breastfed for less than seven months.

Research has also shown that breastfeeding boosts your baby's immune system in ways that give him long-term protection while he's growing up:

• a child who was breastfed is less likely than one who was bottle-fed to get a respiratory illness, up to the age of seven

• there's some long-term protection against gastrointestinal illnesses

• breastfeeding reduces the risk of developing asthma and eczema

• there's a lower risk of childhood diabetes and leukemia if a baby has been breastfed

• a child who was breastfed is less likely to be obese than one who was bottle-fed.

One study found that children born prematurely seem to benefit from being fed breast milk in the early weeks of life: they had an 8.3 point IQ advantage over premature babies who hadn't been fed breast milk. Full-term babies who'd been breastfed for four months or less had a 3.7 point IQ lead on

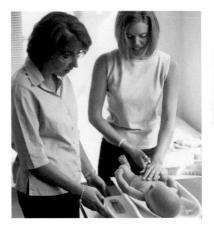

ON THE SCALES
Most healthy full-term babies don't need weighing very often: you'll know your baby is feeding well and growing if he is perky and produces plenty of wet diapers.

those who'd been bottle-fed. It's thought these IQ advantages are due to the presence in breast milk of long-chain polyunsaturated fatty acids that are essential for brain development.

Other studies have found that breastfed babies tend to crawl, babble, and improve their fine motor skills earlier than bottle-fed babies.

Expert tip

Breastfeeding prepares a baby's jaw and mouth muscles for speech. Anecdotally, healthcare professionals report that breastfed babies speak earlier than bottle-fed infants—it is thought that feeding from a nipple strengthens more muscles in the face and jaw than feeding from a bottle.

Will breastfeeding help me bond with my baby?

Breastfeeding a baby is one of the most intimate human experiences: you and your baby are snuggled, tummy to tummy, in a warm and lengthy embrace. It's a wonderful, nature-given opportunity to enjoy being at one with this remarkable little person who's spent so long inside your body. Breastfeeding is the perfect way to bond with your baby.

The love hormone

That isn't to say that women who don't choose to breastfeed don't bond with their babies, or that every feeding will be an idyllic experience. But when breastfeeding is going well, it is undoubtedly a special bonding time with your baby.

Oxytocin, one of the hormones released in the mother during breastfeeding, is known as the "love hormone." Scientists believe that oxytocin primes a new mother to love her baby and to bond with him. It is nature's way of ensuring that new babies are loved and cared for, right from the start.

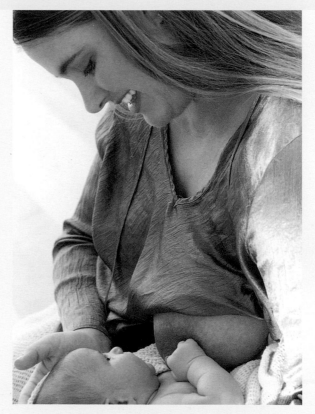

Make time to bond

However you are feeding, bonding doesn't necessarily happen immediately after the birth. Learning to love your baby may take a few hours or days or even weeks. The secret is to learn to relax. Make time to bond. If you're back at home, go to bed with your baby for a day or two and spend some uninterrupted time together if you can. Remember that breastfeeding isn't just about getting enough milk in: it's about pouring love into your baby, too. While you're feeding him, think about how the world looks from his point of view. You are everything to him.

Benefits for you

Breastfeeding isn't just good for babies: it's good for their mothers, too. In fact, just as doctors are making more and more discoveries about exactly how good it is for babies, so they're uncovering new evidence that makes clear the major advantages to being a woman who's breastfed her children.

The benefits start from the first few moments after the birth. Putting your baby to the breast will help your uterus contract and return to its normal size in the hours and days after your baby is born, and will also reduce your risk of a hemorrhage in the days following the delivery.

Breastfeeding also helps you return to your prepregnancy weight—and what's more, it helps you stay there. Some studies have shown that women who feed their babies themselves start to lose weight faster—as soon

" It's wonderful to think that breastfeeding is benefiting me as well as my baby. I'm eating well without worrying about weight gain and my blood pressure is down. "

SARAH, mother of three-month-old Lizzie

as one month after the birth; others suggest this weight loss speeds up after three months for a mother who continues breastfeeding. This is not altogether surprising when you bear in mind that feeding a baby uses up an extra 500 calories a day.

Psychologically, there's a plus, too: oxytocin, the hormone released at every breastfeed, is a natural sedative that helps you feel calm and can even help you drop off to sleep after you've been roused for a nighttime feeding.

And most surprising of all is a study from Japan that seems to suggest that this same hormone, oxytocin, actually makes breastfeeding moms brainier! The scientists found that brains awash with oxytocin had improved mental ability and better short-term memory.

Long–term health benefits

● According to a US study involving 14,000 women, breast cancer is 22 percent rarer among premenopausal women who have breastfed at least one baby than among those who have not. The scientists who carried out this study believe that if all women with children breastfed for between four and 12 months, breast cancer rates could be cut by 11 percent— while if all women with children

Breastfeeding myths

● **You won't be able to make enough milk.**
You will almost certainly be able to make enough milk to feed your baby—according to the World Health Organization, fewer than 3 percent of women are physically unable to do so.

● **It's going to hurt.**
It shouldn't. And if it does, it's because the baby isn't properly positioned. If you get advice on how to position your baby (see pages 30–31), you won't suffer pain at or between breastfeedings. Some women do have a small amount of pain in the early hours and days of breastfeeding as their nipples get used to feeding.

● **No one else will be able to do anything for the baby.**
There are plenty of things your partner and other relatives can do for the baby. Bathing him, changing his diaper, taking him for walks, dressing him—the list is endless. It's true that your breastfed baby can't go too far from you, since he'll need to go back to you as soon as he's hungry. But you can delegate the household jobs while you put your feet up and feed your baby.

● **Your baby will want to be at the breast all day, every day.**
In the early days, babies spend a lot of time at the breast. This is because they have tiny tummies and they're still learning how to breastfeed (as are you). Within the

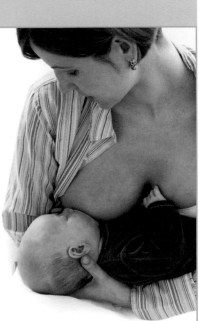

first couple of weeks, they start to change: they get bigger, so they can consume more milk at each feeding, and they get better at feeding. By the time they are a few weeks old, they are feeding less often, and for shorter periods, than in the early days.

● **Formula is as good as breast milk these days.**
It might be better than it used to be, but formula is no more than a pale imitation of breast milk. That's because formula contains no living cells: no antibodies to fight infection, no enzymes, no hormones. Formula contains more protein, but is not as easily digested as the protein in breast milk. What's more, your breast milk is designed to suit your baby—if he was born prematurely, for example, the composition of your milk will reflect that fact.

breastfed for 24 months, the incidence of the disease could be reduced by as much as 25 percent. At a time when breast cancer rates are soaring, and we often think there's little we can do to protect ourselves from the disease, this is certainly food for thought.

• The risk of other cancers may also be reduced. One study shows a 20–25 percent decrease in the risk of ovarian cancer for women who've breastfed for at least two months after each birth.

• And women who have breastfed could also have stronger bones in later life. It's been found that women who have children but didn't breastfeed have double the risk of a hip fracture when they are older than women who have breastfed.

• Another study has shown that there's a link between breastfeeding and a reduced risk of dying from rheumatoid arthritis, and research is continuing to find out more about this.

More good reasons to breastfeed

• **Breast milk is the ideal convenience food.**
It's always on hand, at the right temperature. You don't have to prepare it, and you don't have to listen to your baby's screams as he gets increasingly frustrated waiting to be fed.

• **Breast milk is free.**
The cost of formula feeding adds up over the months and years.

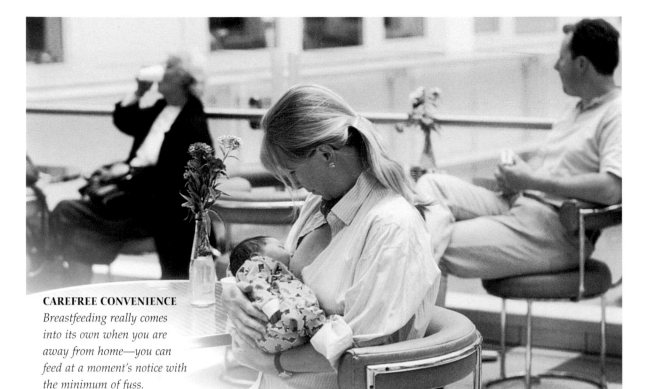

CAREFREE CONVENIENCE
Breastfeeding really comes into its own when you are away from home—you can feed at a moment's notice with the minimum of fuss.

Of course, breastfeeding mothers do need slightly more calories than bottle-feeding mothers, but the financial cost isn't great.

● **Breastfeeding at night causes minimum disruption.**
Although night feedings are often seen as the bane of any new parent's life, there are huge advantages to being a breastfeeding mother when it comes to the night hours. In fact, it is night feedings that maximize the advantages of breastfeeding: keep your baby in a crib right beside your bed, and you'll find you can lift him out and feed with minimal

disturbance. Most babies settle better if they can be fed at night with the minimum of fuss and while barely waking from sleep: if you're beside your baby, with a breast full of milk, in time you won't even need to turn on the light.

● **Breastfeeding has huge advantages for mothers on the go.**
While bottle-feeding moms have to carry bags containing prepared bottles, which need heating up, breastfeeding moms can travel lighter, with just a diaper bag.

● **From an ecological point of view, breastfeeding wins hands down.**

Breastfeeding doesn't use up Earth's resources, nor does it involve unnecessary packaging or waste. In a sense, it's the most "green" food a human being is ever likely to eat.

Expert tip

Breastfeeding gives you a gift in the form of time: time you don't need to spend preparing bottles, but instead can spend cuddled up with your baby. You can, of course, also sometimes use this time to relax and read a book, watch TV, or listen to the radio.

" Breastfeeding Tom is the most **fulfilling** thing I've ever done in my life. I know it's what my body was designed to do, but it feels like quite an **achievement. "**

JACKIE, mother of six-month-old Tom

2

How is milk produced?

A baby cries: her mother picks her up, cradles her close, offers her a breast. Within seconds the crying stops. The baby is sucking, the milk is flowing. A tiny tummy is being filled, and all is once again right in this baby's world. It sounds like such a simple process, yet behind every breastfeeding is a complex physical operation.

A complex process

The process of breastfeeding involves not only the mother's breasts, but also her brain and hormonal system and her baby's sucking.

The seeds of a baby's breastfeeding were laid down years before she was even conceived; it was when the baby's mother was herself in her mother's womb that her tiny breast buds began to prepare for the job they would do one day.

The tiny buds that become this mother's breasts begin to develop as early as seven or eight weeks after her conception. During childhood they are dormant, but with the onset of puberty they develop further until they consist of milk glands, supportive tissue, and fat.

When she is pregnant, the mother's breast activity increases: glandular tissue starts to replace many of the fat cells, and that's why breasts become so much bigger and heavier when a woman is expecting a baby. In fact, in many women a feeling of fullness in the breasts around the time of their missed period is the first sign of pregnancy, because from the moment of conception, their breasts are changing in readiness to feed.

Breast preparations

Another change many women notice early in pregnancy is that the little bumps around the areolae, called Montgomery's tubercles, become more raised and noticeable. These tubercles contain glands that secrete an oil to lubricate and protect the nipples during breastfeeding. The areolae and nipples also get noticeably darker during pregnancy.

The glandular tissues are made up of between 15 and 25 lobes, each containing alveoli or small sacs—these are the milk-producing part of

the breast. The alveoli are hidden deep within the breast: each is surrounded by a tiny muscle that squeezes the milk out along a series of canals toward the nipple. It's almost like having a clutch of straws through which to suck a milk shake out of a tall glass.

From around the 26th week of pregnancy, your breasts are able to

How does lactation work?

During pregnancy, the areas around your nipples, the areolae, get larger and darker and then, as your pregnancy progresses, your breasts grow bigger and heavier. By the time of the birth, the glandular tissue necessary for milk production has replaced most of the fatty tissue that usually makes up the breast, and the business of making your baby's milk can begin in earnest.

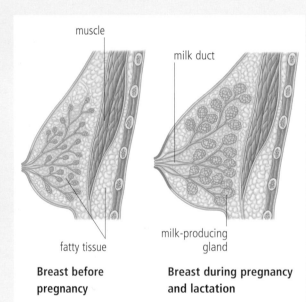

muscle

milk duct

fatty tissue

milk-producing gland

Breast before pregnancy

Breast during pregnancy and lactation

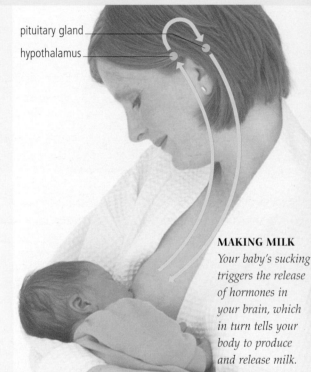

pituitary gland

hypothalamus

MAKING MILK
Your baby's sucking triggers the release of hormones in your brain, which in turn tells your body to produce and release milk.

The process of lactation

Millions of women all over the world breastfeed their babies without knowing anything about the complex physiological process that makes it possible. You don't have to understand breastfeeding to be an expert at doing it—but if you would like to know what happens, let's take a look.

Milk production depends on the sucking action of your baby. When she sucks, this activates nerve endings in your nipple that transmit messages to a part of your brain called the hypothalamus. When the hypothalamus receives these signals, it in turn sends out signals to the pituitary gland, instructing it to release two hormones: prolactin, which stimulates the breasts to start making milk, and oxytocin, which triggers the release of the supplies of milk from deep in your breasts for this feeding.

make milk, so if your baby is born prematurely you'll be able to express her food (see page 48).

Physical changes

• By the time you give birth, each breast, on average, will weigh 1½ lb more than usual, and many women find their breasts remain a lot larger throughout breastfeeding. After your baby is weaned, they are likely to return to their prepregnancy size and shape.

• Your nipples change during pregnancy, too. It isn't always noticeable, but they become slightly larger, and also more protractile or able to be lengthened. This is to make them easier for the baby to feed from after the birth.

• During pregnancy, your nipples may leak tiny amounts of a yellowish liquid. This is early colostrum, the nutrient-rich first milk that will be your baby's initial food (see page 28). In the first hours and days after your baby is born, your breasts probably won't feel "full," and your baby will be getting quality rather than quantity feedings. It is often said that milk "comes in" around the third day: in fact, in the first days after the birth your milk supply is increasing all the time, gradually replacing the colostrum. However, the process does speed up around days two to five after the birth, which often leads to your breasts becoming over-full, or engorged, with milk. If you notice this—and many, although not all, women do—feed your baby little and often. Over the next few days, your milk production will settle down and begin to mirror the amount your baby actually needs to take.

Different types of milk

Breast milk isn't the same all the way through. The milk that comes out first is the lower-fat foremilk. This is altogether thinner, more watery, and less substantial: it quenches your baby's thirst while letting her know that there is something better in the pipeline.

Your baby's sucking stimulates the release of prolactin and oxytocin (see opposite). Prolactin stimulates your breasts to start producing milk, while oxytocin stimulates your breasts to let down the reservoirs of milk from deeper within. The composition of your milk changes to the richer, nutrition-packed hindmilk. This is the quality time of a breastfeed: your baby is gulping back everything she could possibly need in terms of food, and all you need to do is relax and enjoy her company!

Questions & Answers

What does breast milk look like?
Colostrum, the "early days" milk, is yellow and creamy. After the milk "comes in"—about three days after the birth—it will look more watery, with a blue-white hue. Later on, when breastfeeding is established, the initial milk (foremilk) in a feeding tends to be watery, changing to thicker milk that is richer in calories as feeding continues.

What does it taste like?
Put a bit of breast milk onto your finger and taste it. It's generally very sweet.

Does it change in flavor depending on what I've eaten?
Breast milk does reflect the food you've eaten—this is an advantage because, unlike formula-fed babies, breastfed infants are introduced to a variety of flavors even in their milk-only diet.

Will breastfeeding make my breasts sag?
Some women worry about the effect breastfeeding will ultimately have on their breasts, but the truth is that the changes in breast size are most marked during pregnancy as a result of the changes taking place as your breasts prepare for lactation. It's that, rather than breastfeeding, which can change your eventual size.

> *"I've learned that you have to believe in breastfeeding and give your baby time to suck. Then it will work and your supplies build up."*

SARA, mother of Joe, three months

The letdown reflex

As the oxytocin works, you may feel a rush or tingling in your breast as your milk flows freely—this is known as the "letdown reflex." You'll probably notice your baby's sucking changes to deep, rhythmic sucks.

Sometimes, especially in the early days, this rush of milk is all a bit much for your baby, and she may splutter and spill some of the milk as it overflows into her mouth.

Don't worry if you don't feel the milk letting down—many breastfeeding women don't. Also, as the weeks and months go by, you may find you experience it less, even if it was very pronounced in the early days.

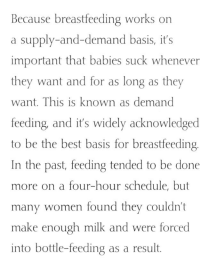

RELEASING MILK
In the early stages of breastfeeding it can take several seconds or several minutes for your baby's sucking to produce a letdown reflex. Once established, it becomes much more automatic.

Supply and demand

When the fast-flowing hindmilk slows down after a while, it doesn't necessarily mean your baby stops sucking. This is because sucking isn't just about getting the feeding she's currently having: it's also about building up supplies for the next feeding and for tomorrow's feast.

While she's sucking, your baby is telling your brain to produce more prolactin to build up more supplies of milk for later. This process is known as supply and demand, and it explains why babies go on sucking even when you think they should have had enough.

Because breastfeeding works on a supply-and-demand basis, it's important that babies suck whenever they want and for as long as they want. This is known as demand feeding, and it's widely acknowledged to be the best basis for breastfeeding. In the past, feeding tended to be done more on a four-hour schedule, but many women found they couldn't make enough milk and were forced into bottle-feeding as a result.

Exclusive breastfeeding

The process of supply and demand also explains why you're advised, as a breastfeeding mother, not to

supplement your baby's milk with anything else—especially in the early days and weeks when your breasts are getting used to how much milk they need to produce.

Giving formula or old-fashioned sugar water or ordinary water can upset the delicate supply-and-demand system and throw the whole process off kilter. Even giving a baby a pacifier can cause problems since your baby may use up all her sucking energy on the nipple, and then not have any energy left to suck at your breast and thus establish tomorrow's milk needs.

What's in my milk?

Breast milk is overflowing with goodness that's just right for your baby. Look at any newborn and you'll almost certainly be struck by how vulnerable and tiny she looks. Infants need protecting, and they need to grow bigger and stronger—breast milk is precisely designed to do both these jobs.

A living substance

Breast milk is a living substance, just like blood, made up of living cells and designed to deliver exactly what your baby's body needs. Amazingly, scientists have also discovered that it changes depending on the circumstances—so if, for example, your baby was born prematurely, she'll get milk with a higher fat content and more fatty acids to build up her body and enhance her brain development.

  Breast milk is also full of antibodies and other anti-infective agents. These antibodies help keep your baby as safe as possible. And for growth, breast milk is not only high in calories (about 70 calories per 3.5 fl oz/100 ml of breast milk), but it also contains a special protein that is designed to be effortlessly absorbed into your baby's system.

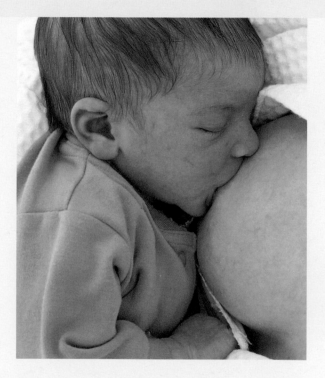

Other ingredients of breast milk

★ minerals such as calcium, zinc, and iron in exactly the right quantities
★ vitamins A, B, C, D, E, K
★ digestive enzymes and growth factors

Are there pollutants in breast milk?

It's true that breast milk contains some pollutants. But so does almost everything else in life (including formula and cow's milk) because some undesirable chemicals are now inherently part of our food chain. Try not to worry too much about this—the actual amounts involved are tiny, and breast milk remains by far the healthiest way to feed your baby.

" Talking to other women who have breastfed **successfully** really boosted my belief that I could do it too. It made it all seem **natural**, and very possible. **"**

NAOMI, mother of Imogen, 14 weeks

3

Preparing to breastfeed

By reading this book, you've already taken an important step toward breastfeeding. Finding out what a difference breastfeeding makes will strengthen your resolve, and understanding how it works will give you the knowledge you need to ensure that your baby is properly positioned and feeding well when it's time to start.

Getting ready

There are other ways you can prepare, too. Talk to the people who'll be closest to you in the days and weeks after your baby is born, to make sure they fully understand your decision to breastfeed and that they are ready to be supportive.

Another thing you can do is to find out where you'll be able to get professional help with breastfeeding if you need it. Studies show that of the women who give up breastfeeding in the early days, most would have preferred to continue. They don't stop because they can't do it: they stop because when they need expert help, it isn't there for them.

Support from your family

Research shows that the two people whose views are most likely to influence you in the early weeks of breastfeeding are usually your partner and your mother, if she is able to spend time with you in the early days after the birth.

These are the people you're likely to spend most time with when your newborn is tiny. They will be there for you, day and night, in those topsy-turvy early days when everything seems new and strange.

If your partner and your mother understand why you're breastfeeding, they'll be able to give you the support you need. If they don't understand your decision, they may make unhelpful suggestions that undermine your decision to breastfeed. In particular, they may suggest you give your baby a bottle—to "give yourself some rest" or because "one bottle won't hurt." But there are better ways for them to help you get some rest—taking the baby out for a walk in her stroller while you take a nap, for example. Just one bottle in the early days may confuse your baby since bottles are very different from a mother's nipples. Giving a bottle will also interrupt the supply-and-demand process (see page 18), resulting in a decrease in the amount of milk your body produces.

Breastfeeding groups

There are various organizations that support breastfeeding women. These are particularly useful for women who are eager to feed their babies themselves but have had little contact with breastfeeding women in the past. If you feel you would benefit from meeting mothers who are already breastfeeding, think about joining a support group (see page 62) and attending a few meetings before your baby arrives. You'll also be able to go after the birth, when having a group of breastfeeding friends could be a real lifeline.

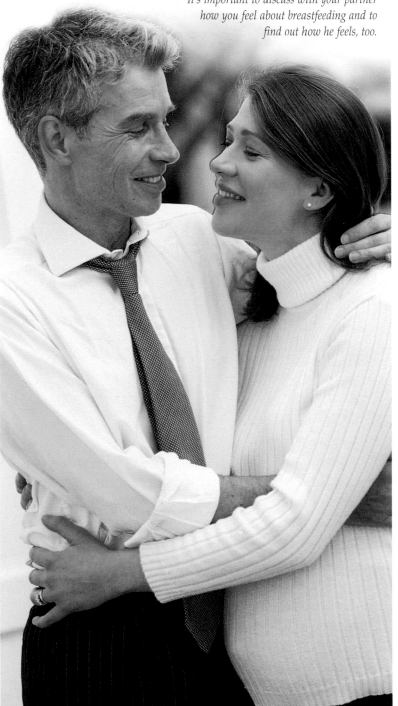

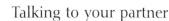

TIME TO TALK
It's important to discuss with your partner how you feel about breastfeeding and to find out how he feels, too.

Talking to your partner

Your partner may not have thought through what he feels about your breastfeeding. But for many men there are complicated emotions and messages to think about. Until now, he may have linked breasts only with sex: now they have a new role. You need to talk about:

● the benefits of breastfeeding for you and your baby—you might

Nipple preparation

A generation ago, pregnant women were advised to rub their nipples with a towel to "toughen them up" before the baby was born, and they were also sometimes told to express colostrum "to get the milk going."

Studies have now shown there is no advantage in doing either of these things. During pregnancy, your nipples are prepared perfectly by your body for breastfeeding, and there isn't anything you can do to improve on nature.

Nor is it necessary to use any special creams, even herbal preparations, to get your nipples ready. They need extra lubrication, but this is provided by tiny glands on the surface of the breast.

One thing you can do is to cut out the use of soap on your nipples from around the sixth or seventh month of pregnancy—keep your breasts clean using water instead. Soap is very drying, and dry skin can crack and get sore easily.

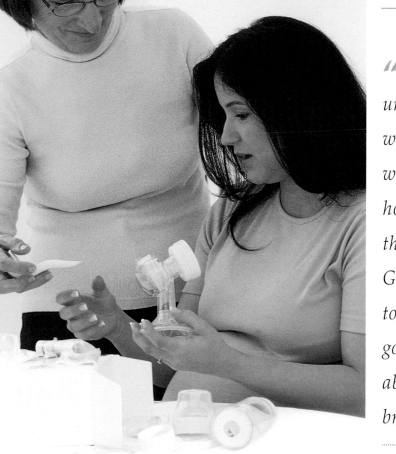

*" Breast pumps were uncommon when I was a baby, so Mom was **surprised** at how easily we found them at the store. Going shopping together gave us a good chance to talk about my plans to breastfeed. "*

JOANNE, 32 weeks pregnant

want to suggest that your partner read Chapter 1 of this book
● the ways your partner can support you in your decision to breastfeed, both practically and emotionally
● how your partner will support you when you're breastfeeding—ways in which he'll be able to help
● how your partner will be able to get close to the baby—he needs to know that there are ways he can be close to his baby other than through feeding; it's important to explain why bottle-feeding isn't a good idea in the

early weeks and how it can confuse a breastfed baby and hinder the supply-and-demand process
● how he will feel about your breastfeeding in public.

Talking to your mother

Your mother is the other person whose views count for a lot. This is especially the case if she will be around you in the early days after your baby arrives. How your mother responds to the news that you intend to breastfeed will probably

be tied in some way to her own experience when she had you and your siblings. If she breastfed easily and enjoyed it, she will probably be a tower of strength and support—she knows it worked for her, and will have every confidence in it working for you.

But breastfeeding was less popular a generation ago than it is today, and less was known then about its benefits. Mothers weren't encouraged to breastfeed the way they are now, and they weren't given the professional

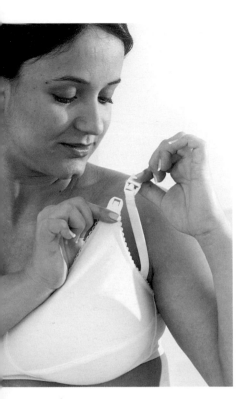

support they may have needed. As a result, your mother may have decided not to try breastfeeding, or she may have tried it and given up for lack of support.

You need to discuss with your mother why you want to breastfeed your baby. You may need to explain the benefits, and you may need to acknowledge that you understand that she did her very best for you, too. Even if your mother did breastfeed, she may not have breastfed for as long

NURSING BRAS
If possible, have a professional fitting for your nursing bras—make sure you can open them easily and that they give you good support across your back.

as you intend to with your baby. In the past, mothers were encouraged to start solid foods far earlier than they are today. Talk to her about this, and explain your reasons for wanting to breastfeed for longer.

Prenatal breastfeeding classes

Attending classes is an excellent way to prepare for breastfeeding. Prenatal classes may be held as part of a course for pregnant women and their partners, or they may be held as a one-time session. The class is usually available at the hospital or birthing center where you plan to have your baby, or it may be offered through an organization such as La Leche League (see page 62). Ask your healthcare provider for details of classes available in your area.

Many classes are given for women and their partners—try to get your partner to go along with you. If he says it's only mothers who need to know about breastfeeding, explain that that's not true; you will need to rely heavily on him in the early weeks, and it will help your baby a lot if you both understand the process. You can expect the following to be covered in a breastfeeding class:

- the physiology of breastfeeding
- the importance of positioning
- a discussion about expectations, hopes, and fears about breastfeeding

Checklist

There are several items you can buy that will make breastfeeding a lot easier.

ESSENTIAL

- **Nursing bras (at least three)**
Buy when you're seven or eight months pregnant—have a professional fitting, or at least try them on before you buy (allow extra room; your breasts will be bigger when your milk first comes in).

- **Breast pads**
These will keep your clothes from getting soaked if your breasts leak in the early days. Both disposable and washable pads are available—washable are usually more "breathable" and more ecological.

USEFUL

- **A breast pump**
Useful if you know you're going to be away from your baby some of the time, or if you have inverted nipples (see box, opposite). Look at the guide on page 49 to find out which kind of pump will be best for you.

- **A special V-shaped or O-shaped pillow**
This will support the baby and/or your back while you breastfeed.

- **A footstool**
This makes feeding more comfortable and helps you position the baby properly in the early days.

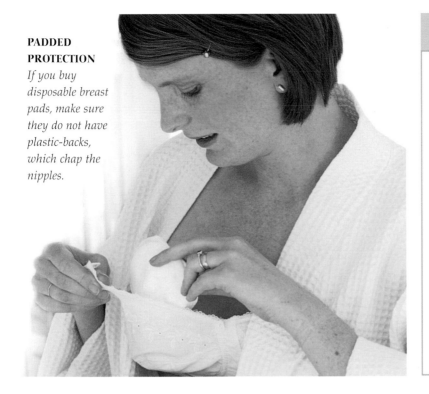

PADDED PROTECTION
If you buy disposable breast pads, make sure they do not have plastic-backs, which chap the nipples.

Inverted nipples

Inverted nipples are not common: nipples that don't protrude usually become more pronounced as a result of hormonal changes during pregnancy. But some women do have one or both nipples inverted, or flat. Check by placing a thumb and forefinger near the base of the nipple and squeeze—if it doesn't protrude far enough to grasp, you may have inverted nipples.

You can still breastfeed—although you may need extra perseverance and support. Using an electric breast pump before a feeding can help—the suction pulls the nipple out, making it easier for the baby to latch on.

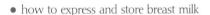

- how to express and store breast milk
- the role of dads
- there may be an opportunity to talk to a mother a few months down the line from you who is already breastfeeding a young baby.

Your professional support system

After your baby's birth, you may need the support of a lactation consultant to help you with breastfeeding, even if you were given help by an expert while you were still in the hospital or birthing center. Before your delivery date, check your health plan to find out what type of

coverage you have for helpful post-natal options, including assistance with breastfeeding.

National organizations (such as La Leche League) and various Web sites offer additional counseling and assistance (see page 62). The important thing is to know where to turn so that if you do have a challenging situation to work through, you can get the help you need right away. Most breastfeeding problems (see pages 32 and 41) start out as relatively minor issues (slightly sore nipples or a blocked milk duct) and getting specialist advice quickly can nip them in the bud.

Some pregnant women know they are likely to need extra professional support in the early days of breastfeeding, and for them it's worth getting to know, and visiting, a lactation consultant before the birth. These women include:

- those expecting twins or more
- those with inverted nipples (see box above)
- those planning for or at high risk of having a cesarean section
- those at risk of having a premature baby
- those who have already had difficulties breastfeeding a baby in the past.

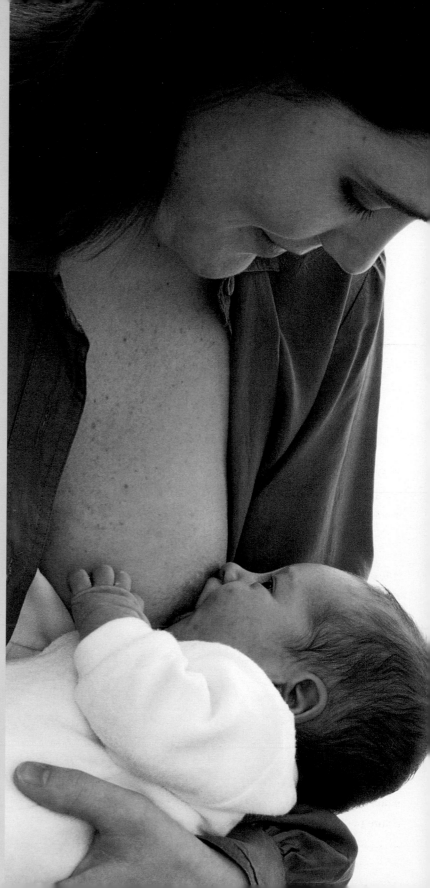

> **"** The first feeding was an **amazing experience**. Freddie wasn't even half an hour old, and I couldn't believe that he could be so **good at sucking**. I'll never forget it. **"**

LARA, mother of eight-week-old Freddie

4

The baby's here: starting to breastfeed

It's the moment you've waited so long for: your pregnancy is finally over, and you're holding your amazing newborn in your arms. For nine months your body has fed and nourished this little person, making her the perfect baby she is now—and breastfeeding her allows you to continue to give her everything she needs.

The first feeding

Breastfeeding is a continuation of the interdependence between your baby's body and yours: birth has given her life outside your womb, but your body will be the best source of nutrition for her for many months to come.

Your baby's first feeding is an emotionally charged moment—you'll both enjoy being close to one another and will want time to savor each other. If the birth was straightforward and you had few or no drugs, you'll probably find your baby alert and eager to suck—research has shown that for these babies, the sucking instinct is strongest within the first few hours of birth. It's as though the baby is primed to start sucking at her mother's nipple right away—maybe nature partly designed it this way to give the baby some comfort after labor and birth.

But these days, many babies are not born after a drug-free labor—and for them, sucking may not come so easily. If this is your experience, don't panic: remember that lots of babies are sleepy following the birth, and most go on to be perfectly good breastfeeders.

Early start

Studies show that the earlier breastfeeding starts, the easier it's likely to be. If possible, make sure the healthcare professionals who are with you for the birth know you want to be able to put your baby to the breast as soon as possible after she's born—many midwives are very aware of this and will take the initiative to remind you.

Expert tip

If your baby is sucking at the breast but it hurts, stop right away. Even if getting her to latch on was difficult, you'll do yourself no favors in the long run if you let her keep sucking. Slip a finger gently into her mouth to break the seal (see page 31), and try again. Remember that although getting the baby's position right is time-consuming in the early days, it won't always be this way. Look at the time you spend getting a good latch as an investment for many months of happy breastfeeding ahead!

Take your time

Don't worry if your baby doesn't immediately latch on and suck with all her might. It's wonderful if this does happen, but it really doesn't mean you're doomed to failure if she

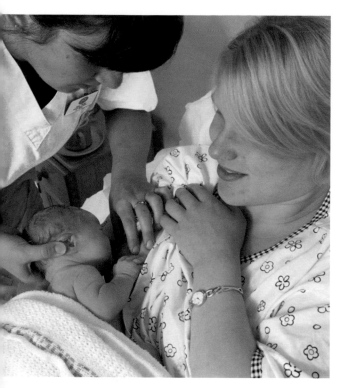

LEARNING HOW TO LATCH ON *Make sure you learn early on how to position your baby correctly and ensure a good latch—this will pay dividends later.*

are trained nurses all around who will support and advise you. The middle of the night, for example, is a time when breastfeeding difficulties often reach a climax—at least when you're in the hospital, you can push the buzzer to summon assistance.

However, if you're in a postnatal ward, you may be surrounded by other new mothers and their babies. This can mean like-minded people to talk to, but it can also mean having to put up with other babies' crying, and lots of people coming and going.

Getting expert advice

It's a good idea to use your hospital stay to get some expert advice on breastfeeding techniques. You may be visited by a lactation consultant as a matter of routine, but if not, ask to see her. And if you have any questions about your baby's feeding and growth that a doctor could help with, make a point of speaking with your healthcare provider as soon as possible after you've been discharged.

Many new mothers worry about the amount of milk, or colostrum, they seem to be producing in the early days—especially if they see formula-fed babies gulping back what looks like vast quantities from bottles. It's true that for the first two or three days after the birth, your milk, or colostrum, won't be high in

What is colostrum?

Colostrum is the milk your breasts produce during the first few days after the birth; unlike mature milk, which is thinner-looking, colostrum is creamy and thick. It's loaded with protein, a small amount of fat and carbohydrates, and best of all, it's incredibly easy for a baby to digest. So, although you may feel you aren't making a huge volume of milk, remember that what you are making is full of goodness. Colostrum is also full of antibodies, including some new ones that the baby hasn't had in the womb.

doesn't—far from it. Many babies are simply too interested in the big new world around them to start breastfeeding right away.

There's no research to suggest that if you don't have a "successful" breastfeed within a certain time of the birth, breastfeeding will suffer. The best advice is to take things easy, relax, and believe that both you and your baby will get the hang of it in time. And you will.

Your hospital stay

There are pros and cons to your hospital stay. On the upside, if you need any help breastfeeding, there volume, but this is because newborn babies don't need a lot of liquid. They're born with reserves of water—the loss of this is what causes the traditional dip in their weight in the days after birth—but what they really need is the antibody protection of breast milk.

Leaving the hospital

In the hospital you may have had 24-hour help with breastfeeding from medical staff. If you've called on them for support, you may find the idea of leaving to go home daunting. Many women, though, find that breastfeeding gets easier when they're back in their own surroundings—it's easier to relax and be comfortable in your own home.

It's important once you leave the hospital to know where you could go for help and support if you need it. Remember, it's worth calling in advisor at the first hint of a problem because most breastfeeding difficulties can be easily solved in the early hours and days. Get help if:

- you have a tender lump in your breast
- you are feeling feverish
- there is a red patch on your breast. These are all signs of a possible blocked milk duct, which could lead to mastitis (see page 41), but with help right away, it can be stopped.

Your emotions

In the days after the birth, you may feel tired and emotional a lot of the time—common problems can seem overwhelming. This is normal, and almost all mothers can remember going through something similar.

Persevere and try to believe things will improve—it might help to talk to another woman who remembers what everything felt like in the early days. It's important, too, to have the support of someone you trust—perhaps your breastfeeding consultant, midwife, or visiting nurse. Decide whose support you most value and listen to that one person.

Breastfeeding twins

- Beware of people who might be negative about your ability to breastfeed two babies. You're perfectly capable of feeding your twins: breastfeeding works on the supply-and-demand principle (see page 18), so two babies sucking produces enough milk for both!

- Breastfeeding both the babies together will save you a lot of time. But you'll probably sometimes want to feed them one by one, to help you bond with them individually.

- A good way to feed both is to use the football hold (see right and page 31). Or lay them in front of you with their legs overlapping, making an X-shape in your lap.

- Use lots of pillows so you're comfortable—you may find it worth investing in a V-shaped cushion.

- Alternate feeding each baby from both breasts—this evens out their needs and prevents you from getting lopsided if one baby feeds more than the other.

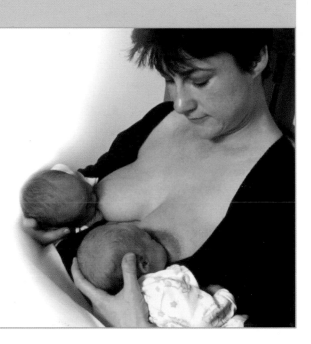

How do I position my baby?

Good positioning is crucial to happy and contented breastfeeding. Not only does it ensure that you and your baby are comfortable, and help you avoid sore nipples, but it also helps the milk to flow properly and your baby to suck more efficiently. Take as much time as you need to make sure your baby is positioned correctly.

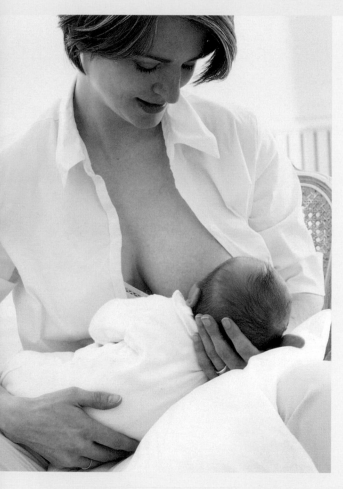

CRADLE HOLD
This is the classic breastfeeding position. Make sure your baby's face and entire body are turned toward your breast—her head should be lying on the fleshy part of your arm. Alternatively, you can support her head with your opposite arm.

Latching on

Wait until your baby's mouth is open really wide before you move her close to the nipple, and always bring your baby to your breast, never your breast to your baby. Signs that you've got a good latch include:

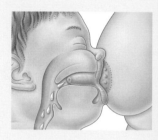

★ her lower lip is curled back underneath your nipple

★ your baby's ears move as she sucks

★ you feel no pain at all or only a slight pain as she starts to suck (if it's very painful, take her off the breast and reposition her because a bad latch will cause sore nipples).

Make yourself comfortable

Always make sure you're feeling comfortable before you start breastfeeding. If possible, in the early days, get someone else to hold the baby while you sit down and arrange yourself. Have plenty of cushions or pillows handy—you might like to use them to lay the baby on.

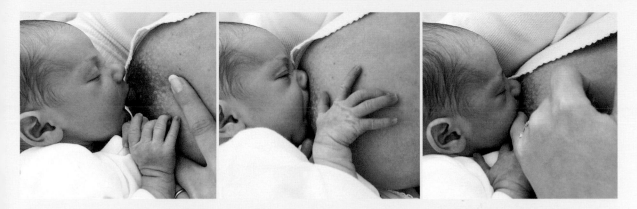

ROOTING
Brush your newborn's upper lip with your nipple to coax her to open her mouth wide enough to get a good latch.

ENSURING A GOOD LATCH
If you are at all unsure about your baby's position or latch, ease her off the breast and start again.

COMING OFF THE BREAST
Slide your little finger into the corner of your baby's mouth to break the seal it forms around your breast.

Once your baby is in position, use your free hand to support your breast to offer it to her. This is especially important in the early days, since your breasts will be full and heavy—latching on will soon become easier and you won't think twice about it, but right now you need to give it your full attention.

Cup your free hand around your nipple in what's called the C hold—this means you'll have your four fingers underneath your nipple and your thumb on top, making the shape of a letter C. Keep your fingers back from the areola, and don't squeeze it too tightly or you may constrict the milk ducts—you're guiding the nipple to your baby's mouth, not squeezing the milk into her.

Different positions
Alternatives to the traditional cradle hold (opposite) include lying down to feed (right) and the football hold (a good position to try in the early days since it gives you more control over the baby's head).

Women who have had a cesarean section may also find it particularly comfortable since it keeps the baby's weight off the scar. Use a pillow or cushion to support your baby's body, and tuck her torso and legs in under your arm, with her head in your hand.

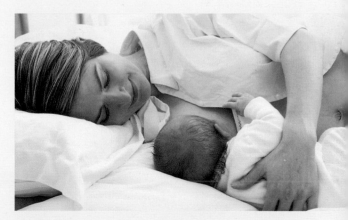

LYING DOWN TO FEED
This is a great way to feed, especially after a cesarean. Lie on your side with your baby facing your breast. Keep her head level with your breast so she doesn't have to pull or reach for your nipple. Her body should be tucked in against your side.

Questions & Answers

My baby is two days old, and my nipples are really sore. What should I do?

You need help with getting the positioning right (see pages 30–31). Ask a lactation consultant to give you some advice. If one side is less sore than the other, feed from that side first—once the milk is flowing, the pain will lessen. Expressing a little milk from the sore breast will also help ease the pain.

My breasts are rock-solid and uncomfortable. Why is this?

This is common in the days after the birth—your breasts are over-producing because they don't "know" how much milk your baby needs. Things will settle down in time. Until then, use a warm compress on your breast before feeding—this will help the letdown reflex. Between feedings, use a cold compress or ice pack to help relieve swelling and pain. Some women find that putting a cold, raw cabbage leaf inside their bra helps relieve discomfort.

My milk spurts out so fast that the baby is almost choked by it! Should I be worried by this?

It's quite common to have a lot of milk in the days after giving birth because your body hasn't yet "learned" how much it needs to make, so to compensate, it's overproducing. Things will soon start to settle down over the next few days and weeks.

Back at home

The big plus to stepping over your own threshold with your baby in your arms is that, finally, you can relax in your own bed with your familiar things all around you. Make the most of it: pamper yourself, and lap up every bit of pampering offered by your partner.

Breastfeeding works best when you can focus on your baby as much as possible. Obviously, you'll want your partner to be fully involved in the early hours and days with her, but also find quiet times when you can concentrate on feeding your baby.

Later on you'll be able to breastfeed regardless of any commotion, but the process of getting breastfeeding going will be smoother if you're able to devote your attention fully to your baby as you're feeding.

These early days when you're back home are sometimes called your "babymoon" period: it's the time when you can nestle down and simply enjoy being together—you, your baby, and your partner. Friends and family will call and want to rush over to see the baby—but, despite part of you being eager to show her off, try to hold back from too many

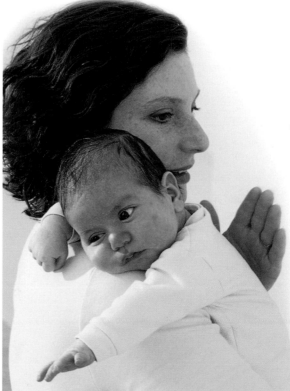

BURPING

Burping helps your baby get rid of any air she has taken in while feeding: a rub on the back or a gentle pat is usually all that's needed.

After a cesarean section

If you've had a cesarean section, you may face extra challenges when you start breastfeeding, but there's no reason to think you won't be able to do it. To begin with, both you and your baby may still feel a little woozy from the effects of the drugs you were given, but try to be patient, because when they wear off, your milk will come in and you will soon become as expert at breastfeeding as any other mother.

If your scar is painful in the first few days, try using the relaxation techniques you learned in your prenatal classes.

These positions may also help:
● lying down (see page 31)

● laying your baby on a V-shaped cushion that protects your scar while she feeds

● sitting up in bed—if this isn't too painful—with lots of pillows across your knees to support the baby.

visitors all at once. Remember that you'll have plenty of time, in the weeks and months ahead, to share this new little person. For the moment, what's crucial for you both—and for your future breast-feeding—is that you take time to focus on one another and on getting breastfeeding right.

Remember to talk to your baby while you're feeding her. Tell her how well she's doing—whisper to her how much you love her. It isn't just milk you are pouring into her little body—it's love as well. And that's every bit as important in helping her to grow big and strong.

How often should I nurse?

It's common to worry about how often and for how long your baby feedings. However, it's best to resist trying to gauge how much milk your baby takes from you.

● Most babies will stop suckling, fall asleep, or just release the breast when they have had enough. Experts do not recommend timing feedings; instead, allow your baby to decide how much she wants by coming off the first breast on her own. Then you can burp her and offer the second side. Some babies will feed 10 minutes a side, others 30. As she feeds longer she will get more of the hindmilk,

which is higher in fat, giving her a feeling of fullness, and she will release the breast or fall asleep.

● Alternate which breast your baby starts on to keep up your milk supply.

Expert tip

It's very important that your baby keeps up her intake of fluids—dehydration is a serious condition in a small baby, and it can take hold very quickly. If your baby stops being interested in feeding, seems floppy, has a dry mouth or eyes, is producing few wet diapers, or has diarrhea or frequent vomiting, get medical help right away.

What's the best way of taking care of myself when I'm breastfeeding?

Now that you're breastfeeding, your baby is relying entirely on your body for her support—just as she was in the womb—so it's important to look after yourself properly. And that doesn't just mean physically: if you're together emotionally, you'll be better able to meet the demands of your little one and to pass on to her your enjoyment of life.

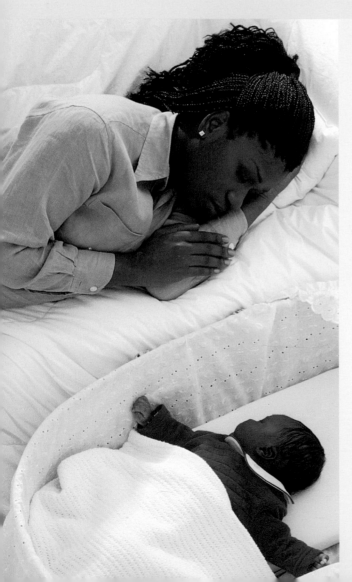

Time for yourself

You'll enjoy your baby more if you have at least a little bit of "me time" to remind yourself that you do have a persona away from being your child's mother. Aim for at least one little treat a day—enlist the help of your partner or a relative or friend. How about:

★ a bath with some relaxing oil

★ half an hour reading a book while your baby naps that's NOT about motherhood

★ a phone call to a friend while someone else holds the baby

★ a walk, so you get some exercise.

NAPPING TOGETHER
It's important to get as much rest as you can—the better you feel, the easier breastfeeding will be. Make the most of the time your baby spends sleeping during the day by catching up on some sleep yourself.

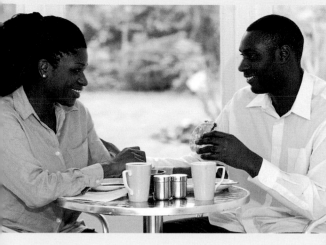

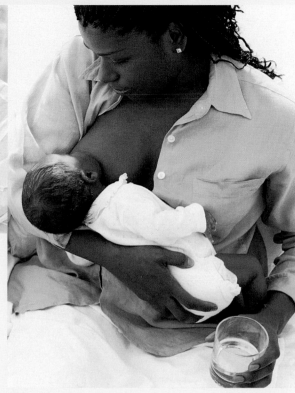

TIME OUT
Accept any offers from family or friends to watch your baby while you spend some time alone with your partner—even an hour to go out for coffee can be like a breath of fresh air for both of you.

Time with your partner

Right now, life for both you and your partner is focused on the needs of your newborn. But you also need to spend some time alone together. A friend or relative might be able to help by giving you some time without the baby.

Your diet

Eating a healthy diet is always important, but especially so when you're breastfeeding. If you are deficient in a vitamin or mineral, your body will respond by passing on to your baby any available supplies; you will be the one who goes without. Drinking enough fluid is important when you're breastfeeding. Try to drink small amounts often.

DRINK AT THE READY
Always keep a drink near you when you're feeding since you may be especially thirsty then. Don't go overboard and chug quarts, though; this alone won't increase your milk supply.

Getting help

You need help when you have a newborn baby. When friends and relatives offer to help, accept gratefully and let them do things you really need done. If they don't offer, ask them to help.

★ Be wary of visitors who say they'll help by holding the baby for you. Holding the baby won't tire you out—making them cups of coffee will!

★ Make lists of what needs to be done so you can respond effectively if people are around to assist.

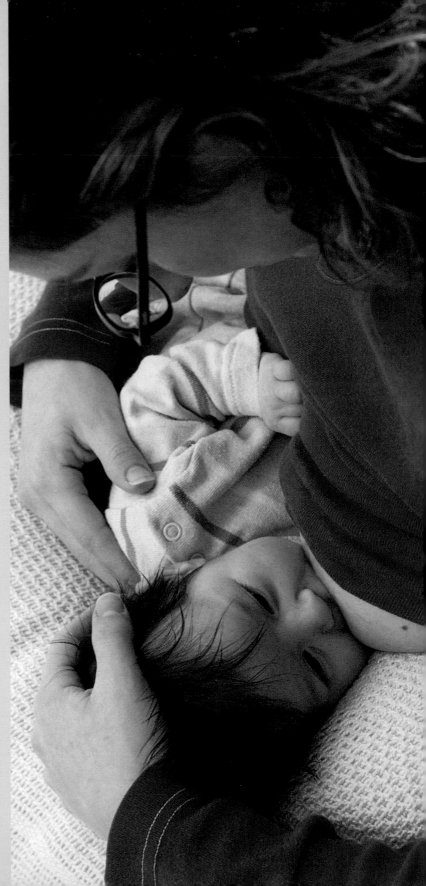

" In the early days
I felt I was feeding
Eddie all the time.
Now he seems to
spend **far less**
time at the breast—
he's a lot **better**
at getting the milk
he needs. "

MARY, mother of six-week-old Eddie

5

Breastfeeding as your baby grows

Congratulations—you've made it this far. The first few hazy days of breastfeeding are behind you, and now you can settle down and start to enjoy feeding your baby. Enjoyment is crucial because with it comes confidence, and the combination of these two is the key to successful breastfeeding.

Every baby is different

For most breastfeeding mothers, the early days and weeks are when any challenges emerge. By the time your baby is four to six weeks old, those challenges are usually behind you, and you and your little one are breastfeeding easily and happily.

Not all babies are the same, as mothers who have breastfed more than one baby will testify, and by this stage of your child's life you'll have worked out what kind of personality he is. Some babies seem to snack a lot, eating lightly and often. Others dig in with gusto and concentrate fully on their food.

Some babies are "fussy" feeders, always ready to be distracted by something more interesting going on—and most babies become more fussy as they grow older, since the world around them is increasingly interesting and entertaining. Don't assume that a fussy feeder is a baby who's ready to give up breastfeeding altogether—it may simply mean that this is a little person with a healthy interest in other things, but who's still perfectly happy to get his nutrition from his mom. Fussy eaters often reserve their biggest feedings for times when things are quiet around them, usually in the early morning and before bed.

Feeding patterns

By the time your baby is six or more weeks old, his feedings will probably have taken on a broad pattern. They may not be exactly the same every day, but in general you will find that he wants to be fed more and to sleep more, usually in the morning.

He gradually has smaller feedings, and longer wakeful periods, as the day wears on.

As time goes by, this pattern will probably evolve further, until his naps consolidate by around the age of seven months into a morning nap and an afternoon nap—one of these,

Increasing efficiency

As the months go by, you may notice that your breasts—which used to feel full before feedings—feel less full and leak less. This doesn't mean you are producing less milk, or that you are "drying up"—it simply means that your milk production is now more efficient, and your body is making precisely the amount of milk your baby needs for each feeding.

*"Feeding Amy makes me feel **really fulfilled** right now. I love the way that breastfeeding underlines the fact that she comes first, whatever else is going on."*

CATHERINE, mother of five-week-old Amy

often the morning one, will be longer. You'll find your baby wants to be fed before and often after a nap, although the post-nap feeding may be little more than a pick-me-up, and he'll neglect even that as he grows older.

One decision you will need to make is whether to let him fall asleep at the breast. Many mothers relish the sight of their baby sleeping soundly, every care abandoned, after a breastfeeding. Some experts, though, caution against breast naps; they say you'll end up with a child who won't sleep anywhere but on his mother's lap. There is no

Is my baby getting enough milk?

This is a common question, and there are plenty of clues as to whether your baby is getting enough milk. Look out for:

• six to eight wet diapers over a 24-hour period

• yellow stools—it doesn't matter if you get several dirty diapers a day or one every few days; in general, babies older than a month will start to go for longer periods without passing a stool

• Gradual weight gain, although this doesn't need to be perfectly consistent. A slowdown in weight gain doesn't mean that feeding isn't going well—it's just a temporary dip.

• your baby's being generally alert, bright-eyed, interested in what's going on around him

• a feeling of softer, less heavy breasts after your baby has fed.

If these indicators seem to fit you and your baby, you can relax, because breastfeeding is going just fine!

evidence that this is the case, and you should make a decision that works for you and your baby.

How many feedings should my baby have each day?

It's sometimes said that the best approach to breastfeeding is not to count your baby's breastfeedings: breastfeeding is difficult to quantify, and it's almost impossible to estimate how much milk your baby is taking in. Don't agonize over this: breastfeeding can be liberating, because you aren't forced to worry about how much milk your baby is taking in and whether it's enough.

Having said that, research shows that babies tend to have between eight and 12 feedings a day, and doctors sometimes suggest counting a baby's feedings over a 24-hour period to make sure they are in the ballpark. Too many feedings, over a consistent period, may suggest the baby isn't feeding as efficiently as he could, maybe because he isn't properly positioned; too few feedings could mean he needs to spend more time at the breast to increase his intake.

Growth spurts

Yesterday your baby was blissfully happy—today he wants to be fed all day! He may be having a growth or appetite spurt, so his body needs more milk and communicates that fact to your breasts by sucking more than usual. This "tells" your body to produce more milk, and it will do so in the coming days.

Your body almost certainly can provide enough milk for your baby—you just have to give it a chance. Watch for the signals: when you see your baby needing to suck more often, make sure you give him the opportunity. Don't offer him a bottle or pacifier instead, or you'll keep him from getting the message through to your breasts, and he'll be even more hungry tomorrow.

Talking about your feelings

Being with a small baby all day long is a wonderful privilege—there will be many occasions when you'll look down with love and pride at your growing child and reflect on how far you've come in so short a time.

But looking after a small baby on your own—as many women do—is tiring and sometimes lonely work. Babies are marvelous, but while you can talk to them all the time (and very good for them it is, too) they can't chat about the book you're reading or the TV program you watched last night. You need other company sometimes, so if you're usually in the house on your own with the baby during the day, try to find like-minded friends to meet and talk to. Joining or starting a playgroup with a couple of other mothers whose babies are roughly the same age as yours is an excellent way to get much-needed company, support, and advice.

Above all, don't soldier on alone. If you feel you have no energy, if getting up in the morning is a huge hurdle, or if you're finding it difficult to see the meaning or fun in life, you may have postpartum depression. Talk to someone—your partner, your mother, or a health professional. If you are depressed, it may be difficult to put things into perspective, so do seek help.

MEETING NEW FRIENDS
It's useful to join groups or organizations to help find like-minded friends to talk to and who can offer you support and advice should you need it.

Fewer night feedings

Nighttime feedings can be tiring, and cutting them down is high on the wish list of most new moms. You can help reduce feedings by:

• keeping the bedroom dark and interacting with your baby as little as possible when he wakes at night, reinforcing the message that nighttime is when people are quiet and when they go to sleep rather than get up and play

• stroking his back or head rather than lifting him out of his crib when he wakes—he may go back to sleep without a feeding, which will help break the cycle of waking.

Is breastfeeding a contraceptive?

As you continue to breastfeed over the weeks and months after your baby's birth, your period is unlikely to return. What this means is you almost certainly aren't ovulating, so you can't conceive another baby. It's important to realize that you shouldn't rely on breastfeeding as a contraceptive if you really don't want to conceive again right away. But it seems to be the case that if:

• you have not had a period
• your baby is under six months old
• you are breastfeeding exclusively, then you have only a 2 percent chance of becoming pregnant.

It's nature's way of spacing babies— your body knows, since your breasts are making milk for your baby's frequent feedings, that you've got your hands full, and stops ovulation to give you a break from conceiving another child too soon.

Some women are happy to let nature take its course if they know they want another baby—what you need to know is that from the time your baby is six months old, you are increasingly likely to become fertile again. However, some mothers who breastfeed go

Troubleshooting

Hopefully you'll sail through breastfeeding without any problems. But just in case, here's what to do if:

• **you get sore nipples.**
Reread the section in this book on positioning and latching on (see pages 30–31) because bad positioning is almost always the root cause of sore nipples. Talk to a lactation consultant so you can perfect your technique. Sometimes a simple suggestion will make all the difference. Expressing a little breast milk onto the sore nipple is a good way of relieving the pain.

• **you get one or more tender lumps in your breast.**
This may be a blocked duct. Nurse your baby from this side as much as possible, take a warm bath, massage the firm area and express a little bit of milk while in the tub to get the milk moving through your breast again.

• **you start feeling feverish or have a red spot on your breast.**
This could be the start of mastitis or breast inflammation. Feed as much as possible from the affected breast, get lots of rest, and move your arm on that side to improve blood flow to the area. See your doctor for advice.

• **your baby has suddenly started to refuse the breast.**
Your milk may have changed in flavor. Are you on medication? Have you been getting a lot of exercise, causing a temporary buildup of lactic acid in your milk? Has your period started again, or are you pregnant again? The hormonal changes could be making a difference. Changes to breast milk are usually temporary, and your baby soon starts to nurse again. Another cause of a baby refusing to nurse can be that he has a stuffy nose. If refusing feedings continues beyond two or three feedings, get medical help.

• **you think your baby is comfort-sucking.**
If you think your baby is enjoying sucking at the breast, but isn't taking in a lot of milk, it may be that he is actually taking in more than you realize. Or he might be sucking to encourage your breasts to make more milk for tomorrow—upping the demand factor. Alternatively, he might just need to feel close to you right now—and who's to say that's not just as important as getting his milk?

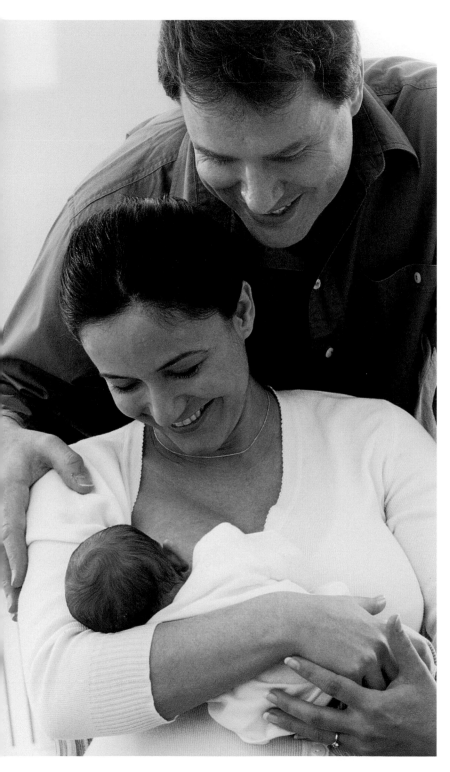

for a year or even two without the resumption of their period.

Most women, though, choose to exercise more control over their fertility. If you fall into this category, talk to your doctor or see a family planning specialist to discuss your needs—the method of birth control you've used in the past may not be appropriate for your current needs.

Birth control pills that contain estrogen are likely to interfere with your milk supply, so the progesterone-only pill is more commonly prescribed, and no studies have shown there to be any harmful effect on the baby. Some mothers, despite this, choose not to take oral contraceptives while they're breastfeeding, and for them a barrier method (condoms or a diaphragm) may be the best option. If you decide to use a diaphragm or cervical cap and have used one in the past, you must have a new one fitted now because childbirth changes the size of your cervix.

TEAM EFFORT
By giving his support and helping you while you breastfeed, your partner will quickly become part of the feeding routine.

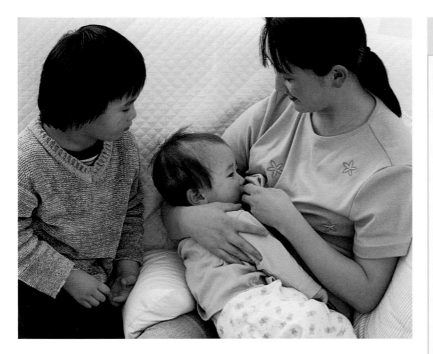

INVOLVING SIBLINGS
Once you are breastfeeding confidently, talk to older siblings while you feed and try to make sure they don't feel left out.

Your partner's role

Will your partner feel left out because you're breastfeeding your baby? The answer to this is very complex: a mother and her breastfed baby have an extremely close and exclusive relationship and, inevitably, some dads do feel left out. But there are lots of ways in which your partner can support both you and your baby. In particular, he can spend time cuddling, and then playing with, his child; he can change diapers or give baths, among other things.

Your partner can also help you get comfortable when you're preparing to breastfeed, and bring you a glass of water or juice if you need one. He can help you recover from wakeful nights by taking care of the baby in the morning, while you get an extra hour or two of sleep, and he can make sure you eat nutritious meals by shopping for and cooking them.

No dad wants to feel as though he's been usurped by a newborn. Be sensitive to your partner's needs: like you, he has a whole different way of life as a parent to get used to. Perhaps the biggest plus for both of you is that you have one another to share the delight of this new little person.

Checklist

WHAT YOU NEED TO AVOID

• **Alcohol** Studies show that alcohol is dangerous for the developing baby. Women should continue to abstain from alcohol while breastfeeding.

• **Smoking** This can decrease your milk supply. In addition, nicotine is passed on in breast milk. Thinking of your baby and his vulnerability to cigarette smoke is a good motivation for getting you to give up, and you should speak to your healthcare provider about ways of kicking the habit. But if you continue to smoke, don't think you can't breastfeed—your milk is still the best food for your baby, although you should always smoke away from him, preferably outside, or in another room at the very least.

• **Drugs** If you need to take prescribed or over-the-counter drugs for any reason, always tell your doctor or pharmacist that you are breastfeeding.

• **Too much exercise** Heavy workouts can increase the amount of lactic acid in your milk, which may affect the taste, but for most mothers and babies this is not a problem.

• You should also avoid caffeine, too much spicy or acidic food, and peanuts if there is a history of peanut allergy in the family.

Can I breastfeed when I'm in public places?

It's normal to feel a little nervous and self-conscious when you first breastfeed in public. What you'll find, though, is that the more you do it, the easier it gets. And it's worth getting used to breastfeeding when you're out because doing so means you'll maximize the benefits—after all, breast milk is the best convenience food ever invented!

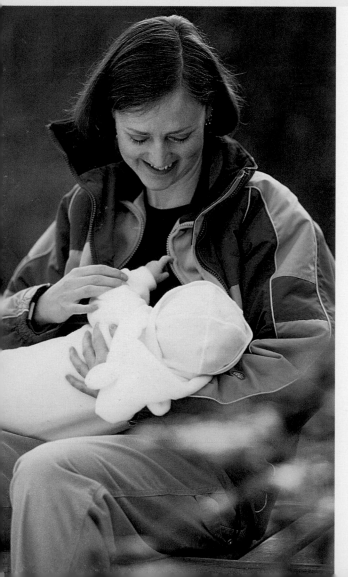

Tips for breastfeeding in public

Get confident about breastfeeding before you do it in front of other people or in a public place—it can be daunting at first, so try to make it as easy and straightforward as possible. Have someone with you—ideally, another breastfeeding mother.

★ Find a place where there are other parents and small children so you'll feel you are among friends.

★ Take a change of clothes for you and your baby.

★ Breastfeeding can make you thirsty, so always carry a bottle of water for yourself in your bag.

★ Wear a sweater or jacket over your top—if your breasts leak, you'll be able to cover it up.

★ If your milk lets down when you aren't ready to feed, press hard on your breasts with your upper arms—this inhibits the flow.

Breastfeeding rooms

Some stores and shopping malls have breastfeeding rooms where mothers can take their babies to feed them "discreetly." Many breastfeeding mothers don't like the idea of being shut away in a little room—

they say no one should be made to feel they have to hide in order to breastfeed. Others feel that they can't breastfeed publicly and, for them, breastfeeding rooms make the difference between being able to go out and having to stay at home.

Baby comes first

Wherever you are and whoever you are with, if your baby needs to nurse, that should come first, and those around you should respect that.

If for any reason you feel uncomfortable, simply excuse yourself and find somewhere you prefer to sit. Remember that the more breastfeeding mothers choose to feed their babies in public, the more accepted and "normal" this will become.

It's also important to know that breastfeeding can be discreet—often those sitting around you won't notice, especially when you become more adept. And as a breastfeeding mother the law is usually on your side if you choose to feed your baby in public. Many people will show support for you if they happen to notice you're feeding your baby: if you attract any attention at all, it's more likely to be positive than negative.

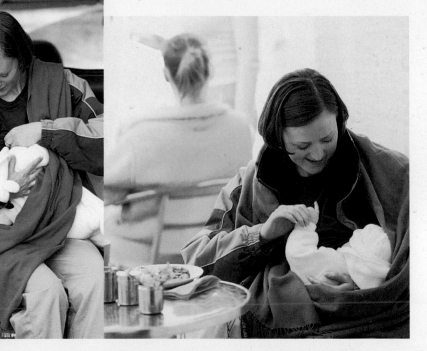

EASY DISCRETION
Pulling a top up from the waist to breastfeed in public will attract less attention than unbuttoning a shirt. It's also a good idea to carry a light shawl with you in case you feel the need for extra cover.

CAREFUL POSITIONING
If you're in a restaurant, choose a seat facing away from other customers—this will make you feel less self-conscious as you nurse. More than likely, the people sitting around you won't even notice that you are breastfeeding.

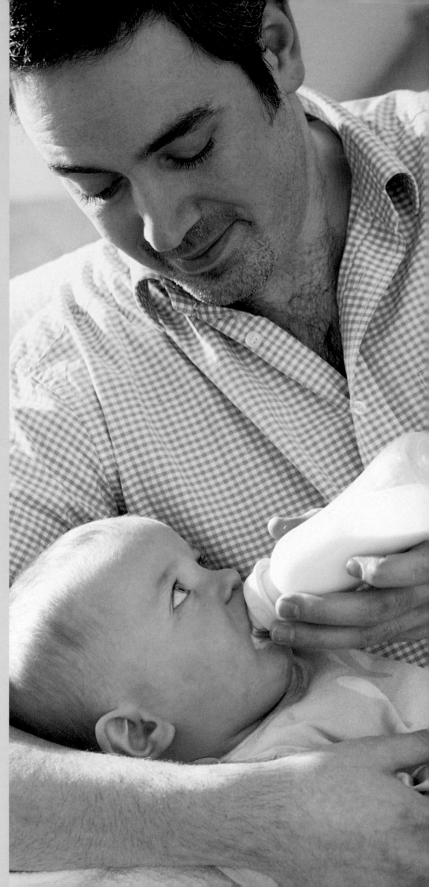

" Expressing my breast milk means that I have a little more **freedom** and time **for myself** while Tim feeds Matthew. "

JULIA, mother of four-month-old Matthew

6

Expressing breast milk

Sometimes babies and their mothers can't be together all the time. When this is the case, direct mother-to-child feeding isn't the only option: if you have to spend some or all of the day away from your baby, expressing milk provides you with an alternative means of giving her breast milk.

What is "expressing"?

Expressing means squeezing the milk out of your breasts. It's done either by hand, or using an electric or manual pump. The milk is then stored in bottles or bags in the refrigerator or freezer to be used whenever your baby needs feeding and you can't do it directly.

There are a number of reasons why some babies and their mothers can't be together. For example, in some instances a baby may need to stay in a neonatal intensive care unit (NICU) if she was born prematurely, or if she has a medical condition that requires immediate treatment.

Another reason for expressing might be if the mother chooses or feels she has no choice but to go back to work outside the home, and is unable to have her baby cared for on or close to her employer's premises. In either of these cases,

being able to express milk, which is then fed to the baby when the mother isn't around, makes the difference between having to stop breastfeeding and being able to continue.

A third category of mothers who might want to learn to express are those who have occasional reason to be apart from their babies—the occasional day away or an overnight trip when they can leave their babies with others.

Expressing milk if your baby needs special care

This is the hardest situation in which to express because, unlike a mother who's returning to work, and who's already an experienced breastfeeder, you'll be starting your life as a breastfeeding mother with only a pump to get the milk to flow. Emotionally, you may be in a difficult situation—your pregnancy

might have ended in an entirely unexpected way, and now you find yourself with a tiny baby who may need to stay in the hospital for a long time, and who you'd desperately like to breastfeed.

For the next few weeks, the time you spend pumping milk may be frustrating because every part of you yearns to be cuddling your tiny baby and feeding her skin-to-skin. But the breast pump can be your friend, too, because without

Expert tip

Hand expression (see page 48) is a useful skill for any breastfeeding mother to master. For example, you can relieve the pressure of engorged breasts by expressing some milk gently while sitting in a warm bath. And rubbing a little expressed milk onto a sore or cracked nipple can help it to heal.

How do I express?

Expression techniques depend on whether you're using a pump or expressing by hand. Remember that practice is hugely important—this is an entirely learned skill, and the more you do it, the more efficient and confident you will become. Some women find that taking a warm shower or bath before they start can encourage the milk to flow.

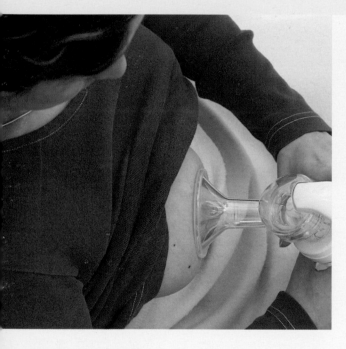

will start to drip from your breasts. At the first few pumping sessions, you're unlikely to come away with more than a few drops. But over time, your efforts will result in a lot more milk being collected.

Hand expression

Hand expression is a useful skill. Wash your hands before you start. Then place your thumbs above your nipple and your fingers below so they form a circle around your areola. Squeeze gently, pushing the glands behind the areola in a circular motion. Use a sterile bowl to collect the milk. Hand expressing is time-consuming at first, but some women go on to be experts and find it almost as efficient as a pump.

Pump expression

Whether you're using an electric, battery-operated, or manual pump, you'll start by holding the cup and bottle attachment to your nipple, ensuring that as much of the areola as possible is covered by the cup.

Switch the machine on or, if you are using a hand pump, start to activate the suction process with the handle. The suction mimics the way a baby sucks at the nipple, drawing it out rhythmically, and milk

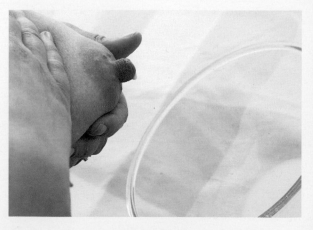

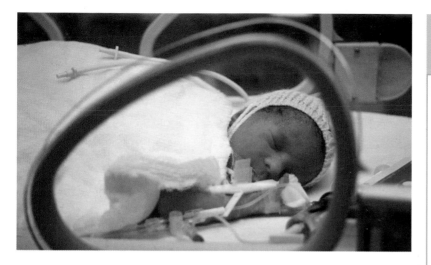

SPECIAL-NEEDS BABIES
Expressing milk to feed to your special-needs baby helps reassure you that you are giving your baby the very best nourishment.

the stimulation it provides, it's extremely difficult to keep your milk supply going in order to feed the baby herself when she's a bit bigger.

Premature babies either can't suck or can't suck very efficiently— they're just too little, born before the sucking reflex has been properly developed. The milk you express can only be fed into your baby's tiny body by tube—you'll probably be able to assist in this by holding the tube during the feeding. Because your breasts are being stimulated only via the pump, you need to express milk regularly and often. Keeping your supply going will be one of the biggest challenges. To assist this, try:

• getting a special "dual-cup"

attachment for the breast pump you use, so that you can express milk from both breasts at the same time— this helps increase your milk production by making your body think you're feeding two babies

• waking at night to express— this increases your supply because your levels of prolactin, which switches on the milk-producing cells in your breasts, are higher at night

• looking at a picture of your baby as you're expressing—this will encourage your milk to let down

• going back to the first breast a second time after you've expressed from the second side, when you're using a single-cup attachment.

Which kind of breast pump?

• **Hospital-grade electric pumps**
Best for mothers whose babies are in the hospital, these pumps, which are expensive and therefore usually available for rent, are the best substitute for a baby's suck in efficiently removing milk from the breast. If your baby is in a special-care unit and is too small or too weak to suck directly from your breasts, this kind of pump will keep your milk supply going until your baby is old enough and strong enough to do it herself.

• **AC-powered portable pumps**
Portable electric pumps provide a means for expressing at home for a mother who's spending much of her time in the hospital with her baby. They're also useful for working mothers who need to express often.

• **Battery-operated pumps**
These are not as strong as either of the above pumps, but they are light and easy to carry and a useful backup for a working mother who needs to travel away from her office on occasion.

• **Hand-operated pumps**
These work by squeezing a handle to produce a vacuum in a cup attached to your nipple, encouraging the milk to flow. They are more time-consuming than other pumps, and also harder work, but are useful for mothers who want to express only occasionally, or who want to try it without a big financial outlay.

How can I store my milk?

You'll need to put your expressed milk in special plastic bottles or in plastic bags made for the purpose. Remember to write the date on the bag. You need to make sure milk is stored in sterilized containers: you can boil them for 10 minutes, or put them in the dishwasher. If you are using bottles to feed your baby expressed milk, these will have to be carefully cleaned—milk harbors germs, so don't overlook this.

Fresh breast milk stored in the refrigerator should be used within 24 hours. Frozen milk lasts up to three months, and up to 24 hours once defrosted. Freezing does destroy some of the antibodies in milk, so use fresh milk whenever possible. But even thawed milk is better than formula in terms of its health-giving properties. Put the bottle or bag of frozen milk into

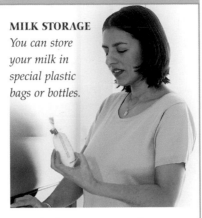

MILK STORAGE
You can store your milk in special plastic bags or bottles.

a bowl of warm water to thaw, or defrost it in the refrigerator overnight. Don't use a microwave for expressed milk because it will kill some of the nutrients. And even though you might be tempted not to, always throw away any remaining expressed milk at the end of a feeding—don't keep it for a later feeding because it may harbor germs.

Expressing if you are going back to work

Expressing is a good option if you're returning to work while your baby is still relatively young— maybe as little as three or four months—and is still exclusively breastfed. After about six months, when your baby is starting to eat solid foods, you may want to adjust your feeding schedule and increase the number of feedings she has when you're together, and let her get by with formula from a cup or bottle when you're at work.

Planning expression

Expressing is time-consuming and can be a complicated procedure to set up at work, but it does ensure that your baby can have as much breast milk as she needs, even when

Questions & Answers

I'm going back to work in eight weeks. Should I start to express?
Start getting used to expressing and build up a good freezer supply of milk a few weeks before you go back to work. Knowing you are adept at expressing will make you a lot more confident about your return. Also, knowing there are plenty of bottles of milk in the freezer will take the pressure off you to produce lots of milk once you are back at work.

My baby will be in a special-care unit for at least a month. How often should I express?
The answer to this depends on your individual ability to produce milk—some women need more breast stimulation than others to do this successfully. As a rough guide, you will probably need to express between six and eight times in 24 hours. Consider expressing at night if your milk production seems to be going down, since this will give it a boost.

How long should each session of expressing with an electric breast pump take?
As time goes on you will become increasingly efficient at expressing, but you probably need to spend at least 30 minutes at a time with the pump. It's worth stopping and starting, and switching sides, for maximum effect. When you first start using a pump, the trick is to go for frequent, short sessions.

you're not physically with her.

Becoming a working mother who expresses takes some organization. Start while you're still pregnant by preparing the ground at your workplace for the expressing sessions you'll need to start once you go back.

Talk to your manager, and explain that while you're committed to your job, you're also committed to breastfeeding. Tell your supervisor that many other women have managed to achieve what you're hoping for, and reassure her that it won't affect your ability to do your job. In fact, many women who express at work say they find it easier to concentrate on their job because they know that although they can't be with their children, they're doing their very best for them.

How will it work?

It's best to think through very carefully where you will express at work, and where you will store your milk, before you talk to your supervisor. Unless you're in the fortunate position of having other women in your workplace regularly express, it may be a new issue for your managers, and it's best if you go prepared with the answers to the questions they are likely to ask. These will probably include:

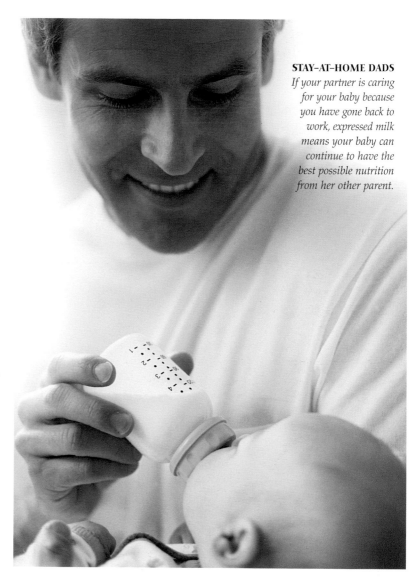

STAY-AT-HOME DADS
If your partner is caring for your baby because you have gone back to work, expressed milk means your baby can continue to have the best possible nutrition from her other parent.

• Where will you express your breast milk? You will need a reasonably comfortable space where you can be assured privacy.
• Where will you store the milk? You'll need a refrigerator—you might want to consider investing in your own mini-fridge to keep your milk

out of view of your colleagues.
• Will your breast pump remain on the premises, and if so, will it be insured?
• How much time is expressing going to take out of your working day?

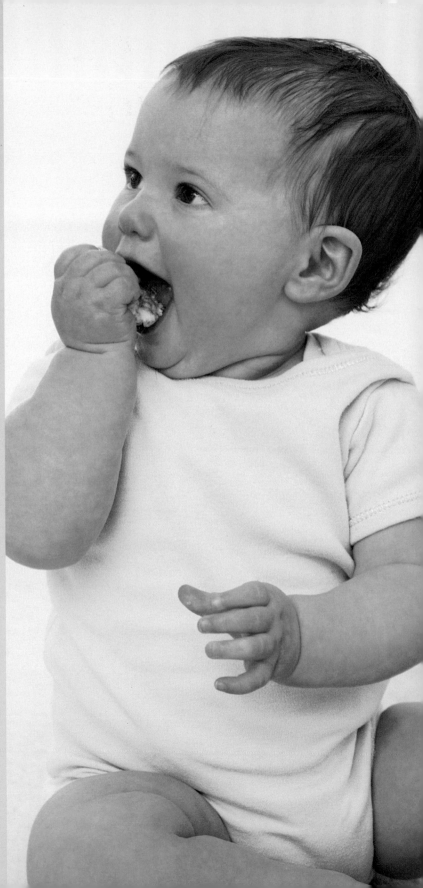

"Breastfeeding is still a big part of Ellie's life, but she also loves **trying out** different kinds of food. She really enjoys the **social aspects** of 'real' meals."

STELLA, mother of eight-month-old Ellie

7

Starting solids

There comes a moment in even the most ardently breastfed baby's life when milk alone is no longer enough. When that time comes—around six months of age—you'll be in no doubt that your little one is ready to enter the world of solid food.

Is your baby ready for solids?

Here are some of the signs you'll be watching for to see if your baby is ready to start eating solid food.

- He shows an interest in your food, and perhaps tries to take some from your fingers or plate.
- He seems dissatisfied after his usual milk feeding. If this happens when he is less than six months old, try to satisfy him by breastfeeding more often—current advice is that an exclusive diet of breast milk is best until six months of age. If you are unsure when to start, talk to your healthcare provider.

What first solids do

- They introduce your baby to the idea that not all food is milk.
- They give him a new arena for fun and games—the high chair!
- They broaden his experience of flavors and textures.

Your baby's first tastes of solids:

- will not replace breast milk
- will not get him to sleep through the night unless he was about to do so anyway
- will not change him overnight into a spoon-fed baby—he's still going to get most of what he needs from you for a long time to come.

First tastes

Many parents see their baby's first taste of solid food as a major milestone—another one of those moments that prove he's on his way to growing up.

In reality, though, the early weeks of mixed feeding are more about introducing him to a range and variety of flavors. Early solid feedings are not primarily about nutrition—although a breastfed baby's iron reserves are low by six months, and a little bit of iron-fortified rice cereal will be a good

First foods

The traditional first food is rice cereal mixed with a little breast milk or formula. It's an excellent starter food, but after a few days, feel free to introduce other solids.

Whenever you offer a new food, be aware that your baby might have a reaction to it. By waiting until six months to start solids, you reduce the chances of this. Other easily digested first foods are pureed broccoli or carrots. You can go on to offer pureed apple or pear.

Wait until your baby is used to a range of vegetables before you start to combine flavors, or to add meat to the puree. Also, bear in mind that there's evidence that babies enjoy their food more if you keep flavors separate, instead of mashing everything together. Offer vegetables before fruits, or babies are apt not to take to the vegetables.

start for him. In general, though, it's a mistake to think of early solids as a substitute for breast milk; they are not a substitute, they are a supplement to the milk that remains your baby's staple diet.

How much breast milk should my baby still have?

By seven months, your mixed-feeding baby will probably be having around four or five breastfeedings a day. However, this is very individual, since some babies are snackers who need several small feedings, while others are guzzlers who can get a big, satisfying feeding from one sitting.

Be prepared for your baby to return to full breastfeeding if there's an

FIRST MOUTHFUL
Starting your baby on solid food is a whole new adventure.

upsetting change in his life. A cold or infection, a change of surroundings, or anything that makes him feel anxious will almost certainly lead him back to your breast, where he knows he'll find comfort.

Don't be concerned by this: be pleased that your baby knows where he's safe, and happy that—whether he has an appetite for other food or not—your breasts are still able to provide him with everything he needs.

Should I buy organic food?

Many people believe that babies are best shielded from the pesticides and chemicals that are found in a lot of supermarket food. This is because their immune systems are too immature to cope in the way that adults' can, and so feeding your child these foods could be storing up problems for his later life. It's impossible to know if these fears are well-founded, but many people buy organic foods to be safer. Organic fruit, meat, and vegetables are more expensive, but to feed a baby you won't need large quantities. If you're restricted to buying just some food that's organic, stick to those items that have a high fat content—dairy products and meat. If you can't buy organic products, *always* wash the fruit and vegetables you use and peel them whenever possible.

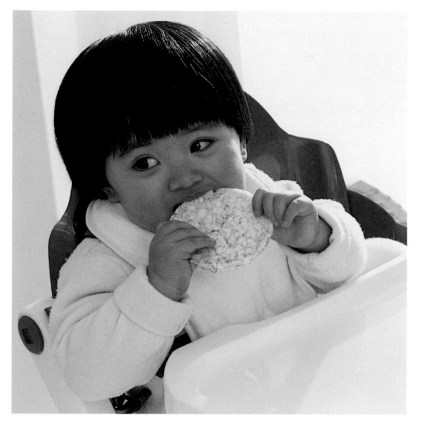

Expert tip

Unless your baby was born prematurely, or has a medical condition, he'll get all the vitamins and minerals he needs from your breast milk, and he'll have stores of iron to last for the first six months. But babies who continue to have breast milk as their main milk after six months may need supplements of iron drops and vitamin A and D drops. It's best to ask your healthcare provider for advice on when and whether to give these to your baby.

Finger foods

Most parents start their babies on solid food by offering rice cereal or purees on a spoon. But within a short time your baby will be able to grasp small pieces of food in his hand and will sometimes even manage to get them into his mouth. Practicing this improves his fine motor skills and his hand–eye coordination, so don't neglect finger foods. They're also enormous fun for your baby, who will sit for ages trying to pick up small pieces of toast or a bits of a bagel.

Finger food ideas:
- "fingers" of toast
- "fingers" of bread dipped in a broth or soup
- breadsticks
- pieces of banana
- thin slices of peeled apple and pear.

Although you might start giving your baby small pieces of bread once he's about seven months old, it's important to be aware that large amounts of gluten, from either bread or cereal, can result in skin rashes. Use bread and cereals sparingly in your baby's diet during his first year.

Make solid food fun

The whole point of introducing solid foods to your baby is to open up a new world of food and flavors to him, and to make it seem like fun. If you restrict your baby by keeping his food on your table, where he can't see and explore it, you are limiting that experience, and if you make every mealtime an exercise in keeping his body and his high chair as clean as possible, you are limiting his possibilities.

Of course, a mess can be difficult to deal with—but lots of aspects of bringing up a baby are messy. Letting your baby touch, lick, squeeze, feel and play with different foods is all part of the experience. Try to give him an area that he's free to mess up

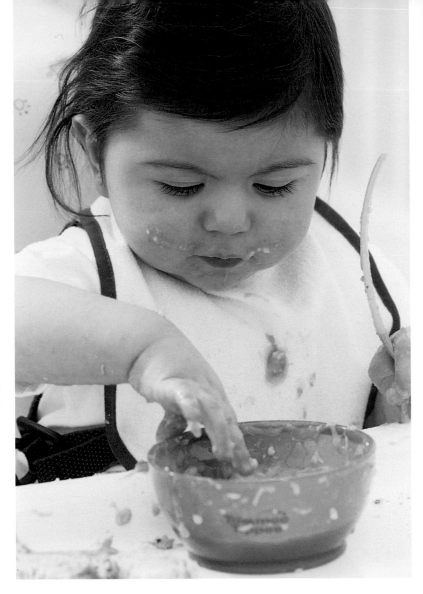

*" They say children need to **learn to enjoy** their food, and Katy certainly does that! The mess she can make at times is just amazing!"*

MARY, mother of one-year-old Katy

during his mealtime—you can put a plastic mat under his high chair, a bib around his neck, and keep him out of range of other furniture he could splatter with his dinner. That way you'll be less stressed about the mess he's making, and he'll enjoy his mealtime and get a lot more out of it.

One approach to mess is to have one intentionally "messy" meal a day. Usually, it makes sense for this to be supper, followed by a swift bath! Some mothers even undress their baby—if the room is warm—for this meal, reducing the risk of food stains on outfits and cutting down on laundry.

Preparing food

Investing in a handheld blender can make a lot of sense at this stage— that way, almost every meal you make can be suitable for your baby. (Make sure you leave out the salt and spices, though, until you've taken his portion from the pot.) Also, make larger amounts than you need and freeze small portions for the baby—you'll be able to give him

better-quality food at a fraction of the cost of commercial baby food. Remember, though, that your baby is growing up fast, and he won't need his food pureed for too long. By the time he's eight months old, a lot of meals will be fine for him if they are mashed—and that way they will be easier for him to pick up in his fingers as well as for you to spoon in.

Commercial baby food

There's a huge range of commercial baby food available, and it all conforms to strict standards of hygiene, sterility, and content. If you fed your baby entirely on these products—as well as on breast milk, of course—he would certainly be adequately nourished. But what your own cooking can give him is a wider range of flavors and textures, since processed baby foods can be bland in flavor and similar in content.

On the other hand, commercial foods are convenient for days when you're away from home, or when you already have too much going on to start preparing a baby meal. It makes no more sense to write commercial foods out of the equation altogether than it does to use them exclusively.

Family mealtimes

Joining in with other people around the table is part of the fun, too. When you sit your baby in his high chair for a meal, try to sit down with him—at least sometimes—for a meal or a drink yourself, and to have a chat. Even babies appreciate that you are taking time to sit with them and focus on the meal and the moment. Mealtimes are a great time to continue bonding with your baby—don't always see your baby's high-chair time as a chance to do other

Foods your baby should avoid in his first year

● **Salty foods:** your baby's kidneys can't cope with salt.

● **Sugary foods:** of no nutritional value and can give your baby a "sweet tooth."

● **Unripe fruit:** difficult for your baby to digest.

● **Tea:** depletes iron reserves.

● **Eggs:** high in protein and can cause allergies—not recommended until 1 year.

● **Processed foods:** too much salt.

● **Cow's milk:** contains too much salt and protein. No cow's milk until after your baby's first birthday.

● **Honey:** can contain spores that cause infant botulism—under one year old, babies' digestive systems are immature and spores can germinate and cause disease.

● **Peanuts/nuts:** whole peanuts shouldn't be given until age seven because they present an inhalation hazard. Peanut and other nut products shouldn't be given until your child is three years old because of the risk of allergies.

● **Foods containing gluten** (found in wheat, barley, rye, and perhaps oats), until six months: sensitivity to gluten can cause celiac disease.

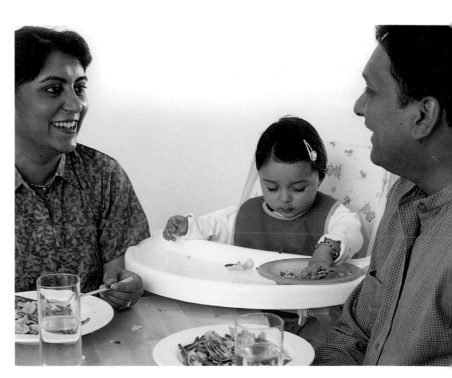

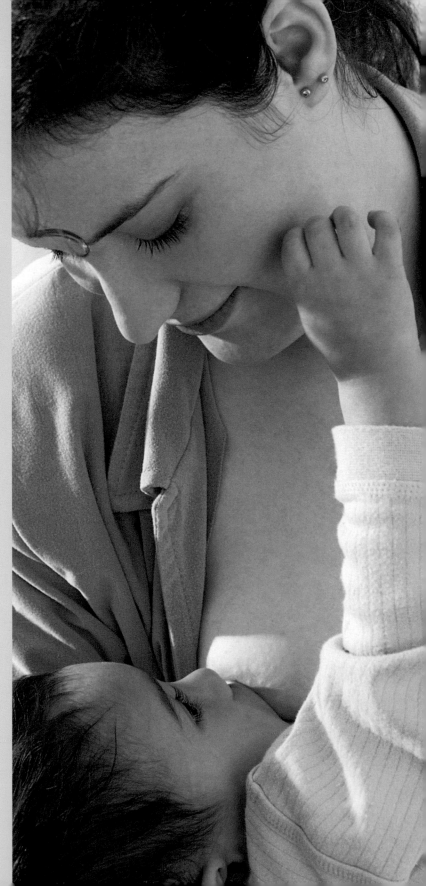

" I breastfed Sam for **two years** and it was a special time. When he stopped nursing, I felt a little sad, but mostly I was glad that we'd done it. I'll always know I gave him the **best start.** "

EMMA, mother of two-and-a-half-year-old Sam

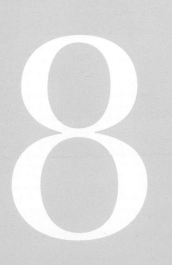

How long should I breastfeed?

Although the American Academy of Pediatrics (AAP) recommends breastfeeding for one year, the decision to stop or continue to breastfeed is up to you. Many babies who are exclusively breastfed, and who start drinking cow's milk after the first year, usually want to keep nursing. Others phase out breastfeeding gradually toward the end of their first year.

Changing preferences

If you have chosen to mix breast and bottle, you may find your baby starts to prefer her bottle as she nears the end of her first year. This is because the milk from a bottle flows more easily and quickly than the milk from a breast, and older babies tend to become more impatient if they know there's a faster option. By this stage you'll know that your baby has had huge benefits from being breastfed.

Dropping feedings

You'll probably find you drop feedings quite naturally during the second half of the first year. As your baby gets a taste for solid food, and enjoys the experience of sitting in her high chair and participating in family meals, she'll often prefer that to being nursed on your lap.

Some mothers feel that by this stage they're ready to stop breastfeeding. If you are in this position and don't feel your baby is nursing any less, or isn't cutting down her feedings as quickly as you'd like, try this step-by-step plan to faster weaning.

Step 1: Skip the lunchtime breastfeed and offer a drink from a cup instead.

Step 2: After a few days, skip the midmorning feeding and offer a drink of water instead.

Step 3: Skip the final evening feeding or cut out the morning feed. You will then be left with occasional snacks, if your baby still has these, and one sizable night or morning feeding.

Step 4: Cut out the occasional feedings by distracting your baby at times when she wants to come onto your lap for a feeding. Another person— ideally, your partner—

Myths about giving up breastfeeding

When to stop breastfeeding is your decision. In particular, you don't have to stop when:

- your baby cuts her first tooth
- she bites you (just say "no" very firmly and move her away from the breast—she'll soon realize that biting means no access to your milk, and won't continue to bite)
- she starts on solid food
- she starts to feed herself.

can help by playing with her when she really wants to breastfeed.

Step 5: Cut out the final morning or evening breastfeeding by changing your routine at that time of the day. Again, a partner or another family member can help by being around

Expert tip

A final breastfeeding can be a difficult moment for you. Far better, therefore, not to have a formal "final feeding." Simply cut down and down until your baby or toddler is hardly ever feeding at the breast. Then, when she does want the breast, just try to distract her, but don't refuse completely if you can see it means a lot to her. That way you'll probably find your final breastfeeding goes unnoticed, because you'll never know she won't come back for "a little more" one day.

to be a distraction. If your baby has a security blanket or a special toy, this can be very useful as well. Try to introduce a new "treat" into the picture—maybe a cup of warm milk for bedtime, or reading a new book, or, if it's the morning feeding, make a big treat out of dad taking the baby for an early playtime.

Giving up breastfeeding

Ending breastfeeding is much easier for both you and your baby if you do it gradually. Give up quickly, and you're far more likely to suffer

engorged breasts because your body hasn't been able to react fast enough to the fact that you've cut down on so many feedings. Take it slowly, and your body adjusts with you.

Weaning slowly is also more pleasant for your baby, who may hardly notice that her breastfeedings are becoming less frequent. If you wean her too quickly, she's likely to be confused and hurt by your rejection of her needs: your breasts have represented her strongest security to date. Abruptly withdrawing them may make her anxious.

Breastfeeding an older baby or toddler

Toddlers don't "need" breast milk for health reasons in the way that younger babies do. However, there's still evidence that the immunological advantages of breast milk continue to be useful. Breastfeeding can also:

● comfort your child when she has a fall or hurts herself

● offer an occasional "safe haven" at a time when she's branching out and sometimes finds the world a little overwhelming

● continue to reinforce the special relationship she has with her mom.

If you and your toddler are happy to go on breastfeeding, that's fine. In many parts of the world, children are routinely breastfed until at least the age of three, and sometimes even until they begin school at five.

Do what's right for you

In most Western countries, however, weaning has been speeded up, and it's uncommon to see babies of more than six months being breastfed. This adds to a general sense that once a baby is in the second half of her first year, she should be weaned—by contrast, though, it's very common to see older babies out in public with bottles.

You shouldn't have to put up with negativity and judgmental comments if you choose to breastfeed your older baby, but some mothers say they get a lot of criticism. In Norway, a country with far better breastfeeding rates than we have in North America, breastfeeding toddlers are a common sight.

Staying close to your child

You'll want to find new ways of being close to your child now that you're not breastfeeding. There may be some special time of day when you can cuddle up together—sharing a book can replace the intimacy of your nursing together. Remember that you won't "lose" the closeness you've built up through breastfeeding: on the contrary, you'll go on building on it throughout the rest of your life.

How does it feel to stop nursing?

Some women say they're relieved when they decide to stop breastfeeding because they feel it has become restrictive and like the sense of freedom and of having their bodies back to themselves. It's good to move on and to know your child is getting older, but for many moms there's also a tinge of regret that this phase is over.

If you hope to have more children, you may like to look forward to breastfeeding again with a new baby in the years ahead. If this is likely to be your only or your final child, though, you may feel a sense of sadness that a chapter of your life is now closing, particularly if you have fed several children.

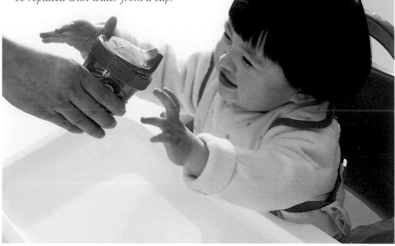

WEANING OFF THE BREAST
Some of your child's breastfeedings can be replaced with water from a cup.

Useful contacts

UNITED STATES

Academy of Breastfeeding Medicine
(877) 836-9947 ext. 25
www.bfmed.org
Worldwide organization of physicians dedicated to the promotion and support of breastfeeding

African–American Breastfeeding Alliance
(877) 532-8535
www.aabaonline.com/
Dedicated to educating African-American women about breastfeeding

American Association for Premature Infants
(513) 956-4331
www.appi-online.org
Support and information for parents of premature infants, including advice on breastfeeding

Breastfeeding Support Consultants/ Center for Lactation Education
(215) 822-1281
www.bsccenter.com
Provides on-site and distance education about lactation and breastfeeding

The Center for Breastfeeding
The Healthy Children Project
(508) 888-8044
www.healthychildren.cc
Offers lactation training for novices and professionals

Cleft Palate Foundation
(800) 24-CLEFT/242-5338
www.cleftline.org
Advice on breastfeeding children with cleft palates

International Lactation Consultant Association
(919) 861-5577
www.ilca.org
Association of professional consultants on breastfeeding

La Leche League International
(800) LALECHE/525-3243
www.lalecheleague.org
International organization offering advice and information on breastfeeding

Mothers of Supertwins
(516) 434-6678
www.mostonline.org
Support and information for mothers of multiples, including advice on breastfeeding

National Alliance for Breastfeeding Advocacy
(781) 893-3553
www.naba-breastfeeding.org
National advocacy group for breastfeeding

National Healthy Mothers, Healthy Babies Coalition
(703) 836-6110
www.hmhb.org
Coalition promoting optimal health for mothers and babies

National Women's Health Information Center
(800) 994-WOMAN/994-9662
www.4woman.gov
Government-funded organization providing information on all aspects of women's health, including breastfeeding

United States Breastfeeding Committee
(919) 787-5181
www.usbreastfeeding.org
Advocacy group promoting breastfeeding in the US

CANADA

Canadian Women's Health Network
(204) 942-5500
www.cwhn.ca
Provides information on women's health issues, including breastfeeding

INFACT Canada
Infant Feeding Action Coalition
(416) 595-9819
www.infactcanada.ca
Offers lactation courses and provides information about breastfeeding

La Leche League of Canada
Breastfeeding Referral Service
(800) 665-4324
www.lalecheleaguecanada.ca
Help and support for women who are breastfeeding

Index

Acknowledgments

Dorling Kindersley would like to thank Sally Smallwood and Ruth Jenkinson for the photography, Sue Bosanko for compiling the index, and Alyson Lacewing for the proofreading.

Illustrators Debbie Maizels and Philip Wilson

Models
Ori with Uyanah Shamar, Hannah Hyman, Erin with Gabriel Sorensen, Sarah with Rudi Berman, Joanna Rosenfeld with Katarina Henderson, Jackie Peacock, Jane Fearnley with Bertie Peacock, Cecilia with Joshua Woodhouse, Beth Biraj with Emma Parma, Simone Alfonso, David with Thomas Skinner, Michelle and Nick Terras, Candida Lloyd with Lowena Bennetto, Michael and Marsha with Nia Thomas, Kim with Carla Rabin, Julia with Lauren Nicholls, Eleanor with Harry Demosthenous, Louise Heywood, Manuela with Ilaria Pesci, Tina with Elena Marrai, Xiaoyan with Rei and Jiawei Guan, Elaine with Emma Hewson, Anna and Andy with Joe and Ruby Worpole, Jenny Cheng, Theo Angeli, Avni, Alkesh with Dhanvi Shah, Teresa Medina with Dylan Escobar.

Hair and makeup Louise Heywood, Victoria Barnes, Susie Kennett, Amanda Clarke

Picture researcher Anna Bedewell

Picture librarian Romaine Werblow

Picture credits
Dorling Kindersley would like to thank the following for their kind permission to reproduce their photographs:
(abbreviations key: t=top, b=bottom, r=right, l=left, c=center)
8: Mother & Baby Picture Library: Ian Hooton (tr); 13: Mother & Baby Picture Library: Eddie Lawrence (t); 28: Mother & Baby Picture Library: Ruth Jenkinson (tl); 29: Bubbles: Angela Hampton (br); 49: Mother & Baby Picture Library: Eddie Lawrence (t); 51: Mother & Baby Picture Library: Ian Hooton (t).

All other images © Dorling Kindersley. For further information see: www.dkimages.com

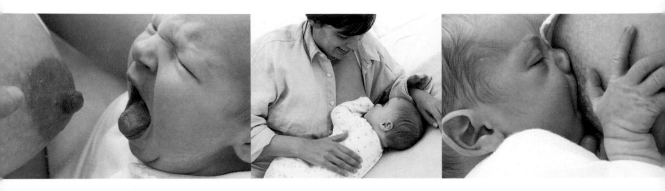